ICD Programming – A Handbook

Eva Clausson

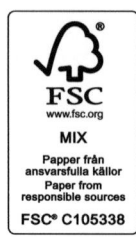

Author: Eva Clausson

Graphic form, illustrations, and cover: Eva Clausson, in some cases with permission from Medtronic

Printing and publishing: BoD

First edition

ISBN 9789174635966

Table of Content

Preface

Every year approximately 382,800 people suffer from sudden cardiac arrest in the United States. Out of those, only 8% survive. In the past, treatment for these patients was limited to anti-arrhythmic drugs to decrease the risk of another arrhythmia and possible sudden death. Today we have strong clinical evidence that treatment with an ICD, Implantable Cardioverter Defibrillator, is effective in decreasing sudden death in many patient populations. ICD treatment is now the first choice, together with drugs, for patients with known arrhythmias such as ventricular tachycardia (VT) and after survival of ventricular fibrillation (VF) (commonly called secondary prevention therapy), as well as for patients with diseases and conditions increasing the risk of developing such arrhythmias (commonly called primary prevention therapy). ICD treatment has increased markedly over the past ten years, from 280 per million people in 2003 to 577 per million in 2006, which puts the U.S. on top compared to other countries in the world. The use of these devices is constantly increasing, resulting in more and more patients with an implanted ICD who need hospital care in the form of implantation, follow-ups, and programming to individually adjust parameters for the type of arrhythmia, ventricular function, patient's level of activity, etc. It is my wish and hope that for those of you who are in contact with these patients on a daily basis, this book can provide you with a better understanding of ICD functions and how they can be programmed. Since there are some differences between different manufacturers when looking at the parameters on a detailed level, it is unfortunately not possible in this book to describe all the differences in depth. For this type of information, I refer you to the respective manual for each product.

Spring 2014

Eva Clausson

Abbreviations Used in This Book

AF   Atrial Fibrillation
ATP   Anti-Tachy Pace, arrhythmia termination with fast overdrive pacing pulses
BOS   Beginning of Service
CRT   Cardiac Resynchronization Therapy, resynchronization of the left ventricle by biventricular pacing
EOS   End of Service
FVT   Fast VT
HRV   Heart Rate Variability
ICD   Implantable Cardioverter Defibrillator
NID   Number of Intervals to Detect
PVC   Premature Ventricular Contraction
SVT   Supra Ventricular Tachycardia, tachycardia induced in the atria or in the AV node
VF   Ventricular Fibrillation
VT   Ventricular Tachycardia

Introduction

The use of ICD treatment in the U.S. is slowly increasing. More patients than ever before are being treated with an ICD, but there are also many patients who could be helped by an ICD but are not offered one. There is no recent publication with complete figures on implant rates in the U.S., but the number is thought to be around 190,000. Figures from the National ICD Registry Report[1] show a mean age at first implant of 67.3 years of age, with more male recipients (72.5%) than female. ICDs implanted for a primary prevention indication represent 73.8% of implants, and for secondary prevention 22.5% (lead-only procedures 3.7%). For both single-chamber and dual-chamber devices, the numbers are decreasing in favor of the CRT-D (single-chamber 18%, dual-chamber 36%, and CRT-D 42%).

---

[1] Heart Rhythm 2013;4:e59-e65

History

By the end of the seventeenth century, successful tests were already being performed on laboratory animals to convert ventricular fibrillation by applying electrical pulses directly to the heart in the open chest. The results were published in 1899 but had little impact until 1930, when American engineer William B. Kouwenhoven was asked by his supervisor to try and reproduce the results. Kouwenhoven, at the time working at John Hopkins Hospital in Baltimore, would soon show that what was described in the article could be reproduced in his own lab. His success inspired others to continue the research, among them thoracic surgeon Claude Beck at Case Western Reserve, who in 1947 successfully defibrillated a 14-year-old boy during thoracic surgery. It was not until 1950, however, that Kouwenhoven, together with his colleague Dr. William Milnor, was able to finalize an external defibrillator for human use. Development of the modern defibrillator then proceeded rapidly. In 1956 the New England Journal of Medicine published an article describing the use of a defibrillator much like the ones we use today. The primary author of the article was Paul Zoll at Beth Israel Hospital in Boston.

The implantable defibrillator (ICD) was developed by Dr. Michel Mirowski during the 1960s and 1970s. Mirowski was born in Poland in 1924 but fled during the German invasion, to Ukraine. In 1944 he returned to Poland to study medicine, only to find Warsaw in ruins and both his family and his childhood home lost. He moved first to Palestine and later to Lyon, France, to continue his studies. After earning his doctorate in 1954, Mirowski moved back to Israel and Tel Hashomer Hospital, where he worked for Professor Harry Hellner. In 1966 Hellner started to have attacks of fast ventricular tachycardia, and only two weeks later he died during a family dinner. The death of his mentor struck Mirowski hard; he wondered how Hellner's life could have been saved. The idea was born to implant a defibrillator that would automatically deliver treatment if needed. Seeking better opportunities to develop such a device, Mirowski moved to the U.S. and spent the next twelve years developing the ICD at Sinai Hospital in Baltimore, and in February 1980 the first ICD was implanted in a patient at John Hopkins Hospital. After several clinical studies had shown increased survival for high risk patients, the FDA (Food and Drug Administration) finally approved ICD treatment in clinical practice.

Some milestones:

1899 First publication on successful defibrillation in research animals
1930 Kouwenhoven reproduces the results from the 1899 article
1947 Claude Beck converts ventricular fibrillation during open heart surgery on a human patient using internal defibrillation
1956 First external defibrillation on a human – Zoll
1970 First internal ICD prototype (895 g) – Mirowski
1975 First ICD implantation in an animal (250 g)
1980 First implantation in a human (John Hopkins)
1985 ICD treatment approved by the FDA
1991 Transvenous lead systems
1995 Pectoral ICD systems
1997 ICD with DDD function
1998 ICD with DDDR function
1998 ICD with atrial defibrillation
2000 ICD with CRT function (CRT-D)

Basic Heart Physiology

Approximately half of human body weight is composed of various kinds of muscle, among which the heart can be considered one of the most important. The body contains three different types of muscle cells: skeletal (controlled by will), smooth (controlled by the autonomic nervous system), and heart muscle cells. Heart and skeletal muscle cells are both striated but have fundamental differences that give the heart muscles their specialized function. While contraction of the skeletal muscles is initiated by nerve impulses from the brain, the heart muscles have their own control station situated in the right atrium, called the sinus node. The highly specialized cells of the sinus node are connected to the sympathetic and parasympathetic (vagal) nervous system, and they use information from those systems to vary the frequency of the heart contractions. This ensures proper blood circulation to meet the ever-varying needs of the body (for example, the need for oxygen). During physical exercise, the pulse frequency from the sinus node increases, leading to more heart contractions per minute and increased blood flow through the body. The muscle cells of the heart, like the other muscle cells of the body, are activated by small electrical signals that conduct from cell to cell. To maintain a normal heart rhythm, all the components of the heart's electrical system need to work properly.

Some of the heart cells also have the unique ability to self-activate if necessary (for example, if the pulses from the sinus node are absent). This is called automaticity and occurs in the cells of the electrical conduction system of the heart, where activation is accomplished (as in the sinus node) by a slow leakage of ions through the cell membrane, which ultimately leads to self-activation of the cell if not activated by an external signal. This safety system may be life-saving in case of failure of the heart's normal electrical system. A slow escape rhythm can thus be maintained, high enough to keep a person alive.

In some patients, automaticity may cause problems when groups of cells start to fire off signals at a high rate. This causes a special form of tachycardia (focal) that may affect, for example, patients with ischemic heart disease.

The Electrical System of the Heart

The contractions of the heart are controlled by an electrical system consisting of different parts. Assemblages of specialized cells in the right atrium form the *sinus node*. This node receives information from the sympathetic and the parasympathetic nervous systems and uses the information to determine what heart rate is needed at any given time. The sinus node then emits small electrical impulses at the right speed, and the heart responds to each signal with a contraction. The propagation of the signal starts in the right atrium and spreads quickly from the sinus node until all muscle cells in the atria have been reached and the atria contract. The atrial muscle cells are connected, allowing the signal to spread from cell to cell, but the valvular plane constitutes an electrically insulated layer that prohibits the signal from conducting from atria to ventricles. This layer is pierced in only one spot by an electrically conductive structure where the signals are allowed to transfer from atria to ventricles. This thread of cells, named the AV node (atrioventricular node), also causes a delay of the signal on its way down to the ventricles to allow for the atria to contract and empty their blood into the ventricles before ventricular contraction is initiated. The active filling of the ventricles caused by the atrial contraction is important for heart function, especially at lower heart rates. When the signal has passed the AV node, it quickly spreads over the ventricles using

17

a specialized conduction system that facilitates a faster conduction than that from cell to cell. The conduction system consists of several bundle branches that quickly reach every part of the ventricles, thus causing an effective contraction of the heart.

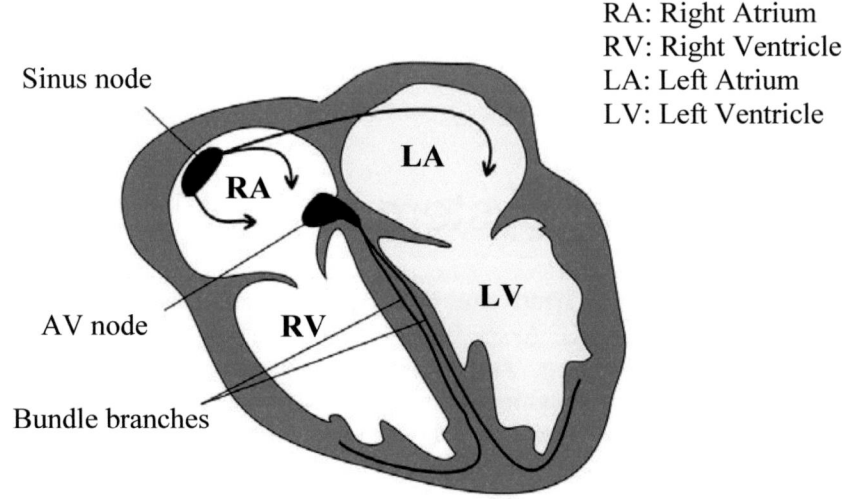

RA: Right Atrium
RV: Right Ventricle
LA: Left Atrium
LV: Left Ventricle

Sinus node

LA

RA

AV node   RV   LV

Bundle branches

FIGURE 2.1 The four heart chambers and the electrical system of the heart, consisting of the sinus node (located in the right atrium), the AV node (piercing the valvular plane in the septum, between atria and ventricles), and the conduction system with bundle branches reaching for the right and left ventricles.

The muscle cells of the heart have a resting potential, measured over the cell membrane, of −90 mV. This difference in potential is caused by an imbalance in the concentration of sodium and potassium ions between the inside and the outside of the cell, created by the sodium–potassium pump. Inside the cell, the concentration of potassium ions is high, while the outside of the cell has a higher concentration of sodium ions. When the cell is stimulated, channels in the cell membrane open up to facilitate an inflow of sodium ions, leading to a changeover in the transmembrane potential from −90 mV to +20–30 mV. The work of the sodium–potassium pump then takes over to restore the potential of −90 mV. This process can be divided into four phases which describe the different states of the cell during activation.

Depolarization phase: A fast inflow of sodium ions reverses the transmembrane potential from −90 mV to +20–30 mV.

Plateau phase: The permeability of the membrane decreases, and the potential over the cell membrane stabilizes at 0 mV for a short period of time.

Repolarization phase: Sodium ions are pumped out from the cell, and the original potential of −90 mV is restored. During this phase the heart cells are in divergent phases of polarization/depolarization, and a new stimuli during this phase may cause arrhythmia since some cells may be activated and others not. This phase falls into the T wave of the ECG and is commonly referred to as the vulnerable phase. Immediately after depolarization (before the vulnerable phase), the heart cells cannot respond to new stimuli. This phase, referred to as the refractory period, lessens the risk of arrhythmias and affects the synchronicity of the heart contraction.

Resting phase: The transmembrane potential is back to −90 mV, and the cell is ready to be stimulated once more.

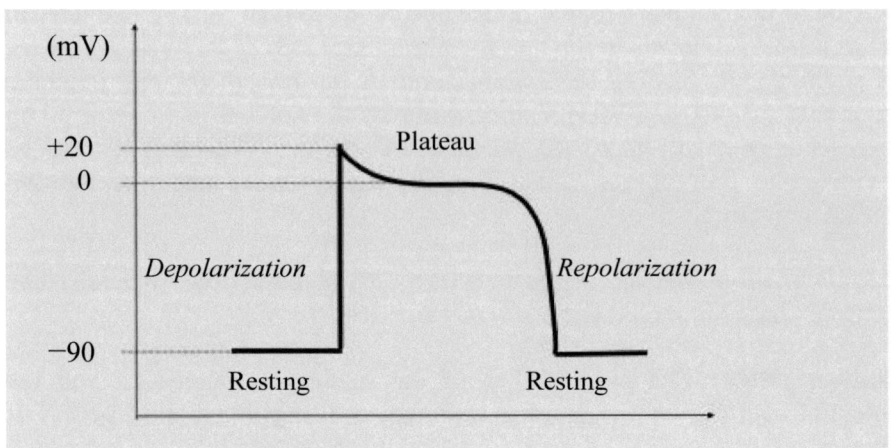

FIGURE 2.2 The polarization phases of the heart cell.

The ECG

During each heartbeat, the heart cells are activated in a specific order. The electrical signal from the summed activation of all cells can be visualized by an ECG (electrocardiogram), where the respective deflections represent the various activation phases of the atria and the ventricles:

P wave: The depolarization of the atria. The repolarization of the atria cannot be seen on the ECG since it coincides with the depolarization of the ventricles and thus is hidden within that larger signal.

QRS complex: The depolarization of the ventricles.

T wave: The repolarization of the ventricles.

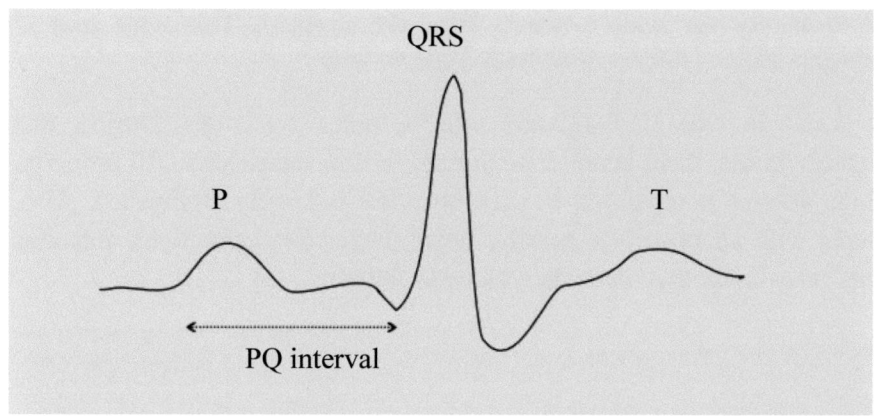

FIGURE 2.3 ECG with the respective reflections marked out. The P wave represents the atrial depolarization. The interval between the P wave and the QRS complex (the depolarization of the ventricles) represents the delay of the signal in the AV node, named the PQ interval. Finally, the T wave represents the repolarization of the ventricles.

Stroke Volume and Cardiac Output

The heart's ability to provide the body with blood is dependent upon various factors. The amount of blood that is pumped out of the heart with each heartbeat, known as stroke volume, is affected by various characteristics such as the size of the heart, contractility of the muscle, etc. Another way to describe heart function is to define how much blood is pumped out of the heart every minute. This value is known as cardiac output, CO, which is expressed in liters/minute. CO can be calculated from the formula:

CO = Stroke volume * Heart rate

CO is thus affected both by the stroke volume and by the heart rate, and it has a normal value of 4–8 liters/minute. When the heart rate is decreasing, the healthy heart is able to increase stroke volume (to a certain limit) to compensate, but if the heart rate becomes too slow, CO will become too low to satisfy the body's needs (e.g., for oxygen). This may lead to symptoms such as fatigue, dizziness, and syncope.

The same is true if the heart rate becomes too high. During fast tachyarrhythmia, there is not enough time for the ventricles to fill properly, and the volume pumped out in each heartbeat is largely diminished. Also, patients with an otherwise healthy heart (better heart function), tolerates higher rates better than patients with heart failure.

Tachyarrhythmia

Tachycardia is used to describe heart rhythms faster than 100 bpm. In a physiologic tachycardia, such as increased sinus rate during physical exercise, cardiac output is increased by keeping the stroke volume steady (or with just a small decrease) and increasing the heart rate. However, when the heart rate becomes *too* fast, cardiac output is negatively affected:

- Ventricular filling time shortens and hence optimal filling cannot be achieved before the next heartbeat. This leads to decreased stroke volume and impaired cardiac output.

- The high heart rate negatively affects coronary circulation by shortening diastole (the phase in the heart cycle where most of the blood perfusion of the heart itself takes place). When coronary circulation is impaired, heart contractility is affected, which may lead to decreased stroke volume.

Arrhythmias are commonly distinguished between ventricular and supraventricular arrhythmias depending on their origin. Ventricular arrhythmias originate from somewhere in the ventricles, while supraventricular arrhythmias have their origin somewhere in the atria or in the AV node. Another way to describe the arrhythmia is by mechanism, of which there are two main subtypes: reentry and focal.

Ventricular Tachyarrhythmia (VT)

Arrhythmias that originate, and are sustained, in the ventricles are called ventricular arrhythmias, or VT. Ventricular tachycardia may be divided into different groups depending on the mechanism behind the arrhythmia. We differentiate between monomorphic and polymorphic tachycardia, where the monomorphic presents complexes of only one morphology on surface ECG (same polarization pattern), while the polymorphic presents complexes of varying morphology (a more chaotic ventricular activation). Different arrhythmias call for different treatment strategies. An ICD may be programmed to a number of therapies to adapt to the individual patient's need. To be able to choose an appropriate therapy, a short description of the more common arrhythmias and their therapies can be found below.

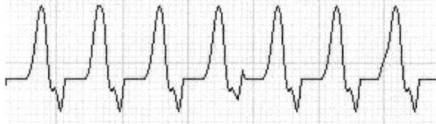 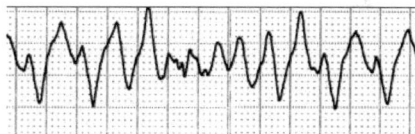

FIGURE 2.4 Left: monomorphic VT where each signal is of the same morphology. Right: polymorphic VT where the morphology of the individual signals is not the same.

Reentry Tachycardia

The most common form of tachycardia is reentry tachycardia. This arrhythmia occurs when the depolarization wave front gets caught in a loop over the heart tissue. This may happen when there are dual, parallel conduction paths that have different conduction characteristics and that conduct around a central conduction block. This block may consist of, for example, scar tissue from a previous infarction or other types of tissue damage due to heart disease. The pathways must be connected at both ends and have very specific characteristics. The first pathway must have fast conduction (speed) and a long refractory time (slow recovery), while the second pathway should reverse that behavior with slow conduction but a shorter refractory time. With this so-called substrate for arrhythmia in the myocardium, the depolarization signal from a premature ventricular beat may follow both pathways in parallel until, in the fast pathway (with a long refractory time), it reaches refractory tissue from the previous contraction and is extinguished. However, the signal fraction that follows the slow conduction pathway continues until it reaches the fast pathway, now recovered from refractory, and conducts "backwards" toward its starting point. In this way a loop is formed in the ventricular myocardium, which leads to a tachycardia with monomorphic complexes. Reentry tachycardia can often be terminated by ATP (anti-tachy pace) without the need for high-voltage shock therapy.

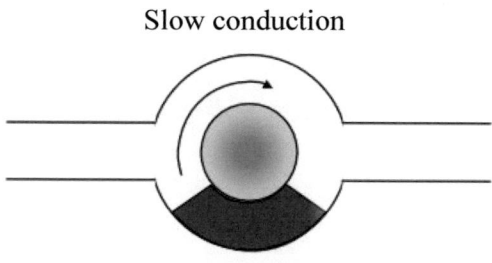

Slow conduction

Long refractory time

FIGURE 2.5 Reentry circuit where the polarization circulates around a central conduction block.

To distinguish a reentry tachycardia from a focal tachycardia (see below), an electrophysiologic study with stimulated extra systoles may be performed. The way in which the signals spread during the induced tachycardia will tell whether the arrhythmia is of reentry or focal type. If the arrhythmia is of reentry type, ICD treatment with ATP therapy is usually successful, although this therapy is less successful in focal arrhythmias.

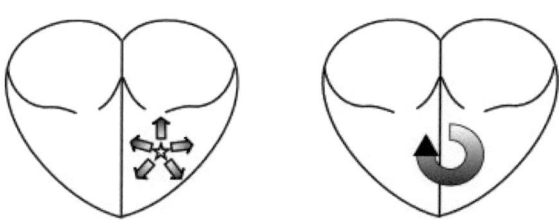

FIGURE 2.6 Substrate for tachycardia. Left: focal substrate spreading from one point. Right: reentry circuit with a circular depolarization wave around a central block.

Focal Ventricular Tachycardia

While reentry tachycardia is seldom seen in patients with structurally normal hearts, focal arrhythmias may be found in patients even without structural heart disease. As opposed to reentry tachycardia, focal tachycardia starts at a specific point (focus) and spreads out equally from this point in all directions. Focal tachycardia may be caused by triggered activity, automaticity, or micro-reentry. However, it is not an easy task, even during an electrophysiologic study, to differentiate a reentry tachycardia from a focal one. Focal arrhythmias with triggered activity arise due to an early after depolarization, and are commonly thought to be the mechanism behind Torsade de pointes in long QT syndrome. Arrhythmias initiated by triggered activity may be initiated and terminated with different stimulation protocols (ATP), but the same is not true for focal arrhythmias initiated by automaticity (through spontaneous depolarization at the end of the action potential). Focal arrhythmias are today treated successfully with ablation.

Ventricular Fibrillation

Ventricular fibrillation (VF) is the most common cause of sudden cardiac death. The electrical activity of the ventricular cells is chaotic (disorganized), and the heart muscle does not contract in an organized manner, resulting in an immediate circulatory collapse. VF can only be terminated by high-voltage shock therapy.

There are several reasons why VF may initiate—for example, acute myocardial infarction, degenerating VT, long QT syndrome, Brugada syndrome, and WPW with uncontrolled ventricular rhythm during atrial fibrillation.

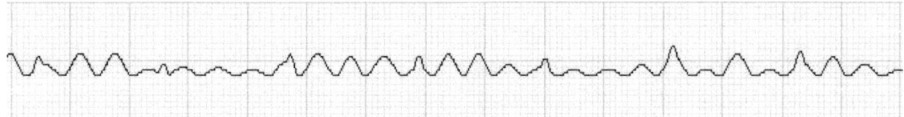

FIGURE 2.7 ECG demonstrating ventricular fibrillation (VF)

Supraventricular Tachycardia

Arrhythmias that originate above the ventricles are called supraventricular (SVT). They may originate in the atria, in the pulmonary veins, or in the AV node, and may cause problems in ICD treatment if the resulting ventricular rate falls within the programmed detection zone for arrhythmia. As with VT, the mechanisms for SVT may be of focal or reentry type.

Some ICDs offer the possibility to treat atrial tachyarrhythmia also, most commonly by ATP. During the early twenty-first century, some patients with difficult-to-convert atrial fibrillation were implanted with devices for internal, automatic cardioversion. However, this treatment was never fully accepted since high-voltage therapy is perceived as very painful, even at low energies.

Atrial Flutter

Atrial flutter is a reentry tachycardia that is characterized on surface ECG by a saw-tooth pattern representing the atrial signals, with a rate of approximately 220–350 bpm. It is difficult to find an isoelectric baseline in atrial flutter, and the T waves are hidden in the flutter waves. Ventricular response to the fast atrial rhythm may vary with the conductivity of the AV node. 2:1 or 4:1 block is commonly seen, together with a regular ventricular rate and narrow QRSs.

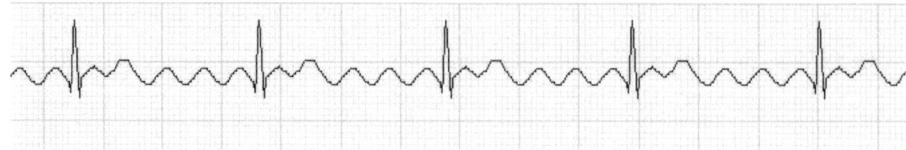

FIGURE 2.8 ECG demonstrating atrial flutter. Note the saw-tooth pattern representing atrial depolarization.

Atrial Fibrillation

Atrial fibrillation is the most common arrhythmia, with a prevalence of approximately 1% for the general population, increasing to approximately 10% for individuals above 80 years of age. The underlying cause is not always known, and atrial fibrillation may be triggered by many different factors. The electrical signal conduction is chaotic, often with several smaller reentry circuits. The ventricular rate is limited only by the AV nodal conductivity and, if left untreated, may reach 120–200 bpm. QRS complexes are narrow since the signals are spread via the conduction system, but the rhythm at rest is often highly irregular. Absence of P waves on surface ECG and an oscillating baseline are common characteristics. During atrial fibrillation, no atrial contraction takes place, leading to compromised stroke volume and cardiac output.

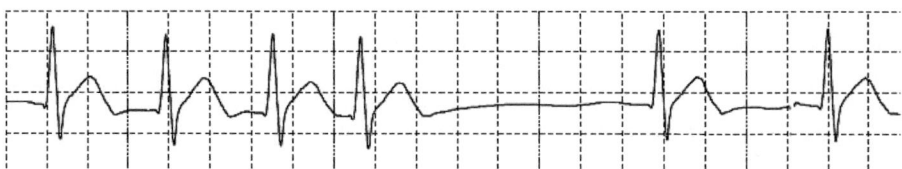

FIGURE 2.9 ECG demonstrating atrial fibrillation. Note the lack of P waves and the irregular ventricular rhythm.

AVNRT

AV nodal reentry tachycardia is a type of reentry where the whole reentry circuit can be found in the AV node. This is a rather common supraventricular arrhythmia that may affect patients with dual AV pathways. The tachycardia rate is commonly 150–230 bpm and RP time (from ventricle to atrium) is typically < 70 ms. AVNRT may today be successfully ablated.

Other SVT

Atrial arrhythmias may also be divided into focal or reentry type. Whether ATP therapy can be used successfully to terminate the arrhythmia is highly dependent on the substrate.

WPW and Accessory Pathways

Yet another type of arrhythmia may be seen in patients with accessory pathways between atrium and ventricle. Normally the AV node is the only electrical connection between atrium and ventricle, but in some patients one or more extra pathways exist. A special type of reentry may then develop that involves both atria and ventricles, using the AV node and the accessory pathway for conduction in different directions. Depending on how the depolarization is spread, these arrhythmias are divided into orthodromic and antidromic types. Orthodromic arrhythmia is more common and is characterized by antegrade (A to V) conduction over the AV node and retrograde (V to A) conduction over the accessory pathway. Hence, AV conduction is performed over the AV node, leading to narrow QRSs. Antidromic arrhythmias conduct in the reversed direction, i.e., retrograde conduction over the AV node and antegrade conduction over the accessory pathway, almost always resulting in broad QRSs (unless the accessory pathway is situated very close to the AV node). Patients with accessory pathways are today completely cured if successfully treated with ablation. ICD is not an option.

Orthodromic   Antidromic

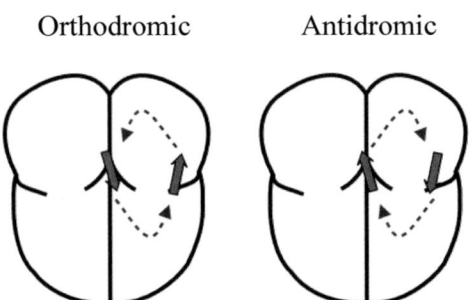

FIGURE 2.10 Left: orthodromic tachycardia with antegrade (AV) conduction over the AV node. Right: antidromic tachycardia with retrograde (VA) conduction over the AV node.

Wolff–Parkinson–White (WPW) Syndrome

This is the most common AV reentry tachycardia, and is made possible through pre-excitation of an accessory pathway called Kent's bundle. This bundle lacks the decremental properties of the AV node and hence conducts at a faster speed. On surface ECG a short PQ interval may be seen (< 120 ms), together with broad QRSs (since Kent's bundle is discharged not into the conduction system but in the more slowly conducting ventricular muscle cells). During sinus rhythm, the start of the QRS is found very close to the P wave, demonstrating a so-called delta wave on surface ECG. However, the atrial signal also conducts over the AV node and reaches the ventricles somewhat later due to its delaying properties. When the signal from the AV node reaches the ventricles, it is quickly spread over the rest of the myocardium using the conduction system, resulting in a narrow QRS complex that is found "on top" of the overall QRS at the end (see figure below). The delta wave is typical in WPW syndrome. There is, however, also another WPW type, called concealed WPW, where the accessory pathway only conducts in the retrograde direction. In this type, no delta waves are found during sinus rhythm. Tachycardia in WPW syndrome is most commonly orthodromic with narrow QRSs. Fewer than 10% are antidromic. Today the accessory pathway may be successfully ablated, and these patients are not candidates for an ICD.

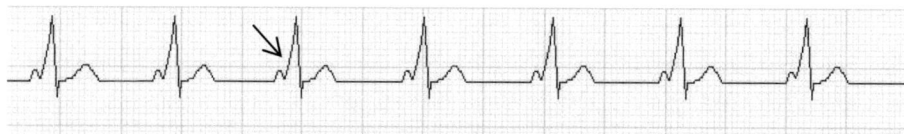

FIGURE 2.11 ECG demonstrating delta waves in WPW syndrome. Note the early start of the R wave, directly after the P wave, marked with an arrow.

Defibrillation Theory

Whether defibrillation is successful or not depends on many different factors, among which one is probabilistic (by chance). This makes it impossible to foresee the outcome of an individual defibrillation therapy. Factors affecting the outcome include:

- The energy of the defibrillation pulse
- The characteristics of the defibrillation pulse
- Lead design and position in the heart
- Energy density on the lead's electrical electrodes
- Amount of ventricular cells depolarized by the pulse
- Defibrillation threshold (affected by anti-arrhythmic drugs, ion concentrations, cardiac muscle oxygenation, time in VF, etc.)
- The probabilistic component of VF

Defibrillation Threshold (DFT)

The defibrillation threshold (DFT) is defined as the amount of energy (in Joules, J) necessary at any given moment to convert an ongoing ventricular fibrillation. The defibrillation threshold, unlike the pacing threshold, is probabilistic. A high-voltage pulse with enough energy to convert VF once in a patient may very well fail to do so in a new, seemingly similar attempt in the same patient. Hence, the DFT cannot be seen as a definite value. A patient with a low DFT is a patient in whom it is possible to convert VF with only a low amount of energy most of the time. In such a patient, occasional failures to convert may be seen, even with higher energy pulses. It is therefore not possible to determine the probability of repeated successful defibrillation by inducing VF once and delivering only one defibrillation pulse, even if it is successful and of low energy. If we induce VF and the ICD is not successful at converting it, we cannot know whether the DFT is high or whether it was a random failure simply due to chance. To know the difference, we would have to repeatedly induce VF and let the ICD try to convert it.

DFT is also affected by the patient's medical status at the time of VF. It is not very likely that this is the same when a clinical arrhythmia initiates outside the hospital as it is during surgery, when the patient is carefully managed. Many factors may play a role, and the practice of mandatory induction of VF during implant is debated. Induction of VF is always a risk to the patient, with the risk increasing as heart function diminishes. Although the clinical benefit of induction may be discussed, the technical check of system integrity is missed if the ICD is not allowed to deliver high energy therapy. Were all connections correctly made? Is sensing working properly even during VF? It is possible that one should also consider that available clinical evidence for ICD treatment is based on studies where induction was part of the protocol.

The Defibrillation Pulse

The maximum energy that the ICD can deliver depends on the model and manufacturer. Most commonly seen today is a maximum energy of 35 Joules (J). In order to deliver this energy during the 1–3-ms-long pulse (depending on the high-voltage impedance of the lead), a voltage of 750–800 V is needed!

Tilt

Older ICD systems, as well as older external defibrillators, used a so-called monophasic defibrillation pulse. Research has shown that the DFT may be decreased if the pulse is given in a biphasic manner instead, meaning that the energy is delivered as two pulses directly after each other, the latter of which is delivered with reversed polarity. This pulse type is therefore used in modern ICDs. The relation between the two pulses is called tilt. At 50% tilt, half of the programmed energy is delivered in pulse one. After reversing the pulse polarity, 50% of the remaining energy in the capacitor is delivered in the second pulse.

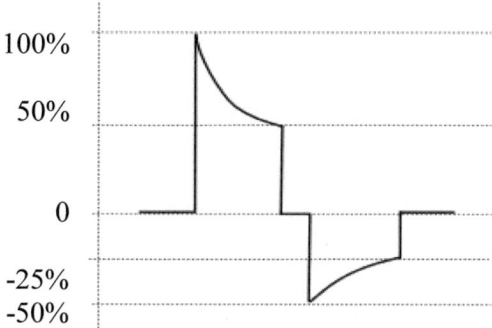

FIGURE 3.1 The biphasic defibrillation pulse at 50% tilt. When 50% of the energy in the capacitor has been delivered, the pulse polarity is switched and energy is delivered with reversed polarity until 25% of capacitor energy is left, which is when the energy delivery stops.

When using dual-coil defibrillation leads, a 50% tilt has been shown to result in a slightly lower DFT than a tilt of 65%.[2] Some manufacturers offer the possibility to program tilt, or alternatively pulse width (which directly influences the tilt). Since DFT is probabilistic, as described earlier, it is very difficult to prove that a change of tilt/pulse width during induction and defibrillation has a positive effect. On top of this, the amount of energy delivered is affected by the tilt, where a change of tilt may lead to less energy being delivered. A 50% tilt is thought to be optimal for most clinical situations.

---

[2] PACE 2001;24:60-5

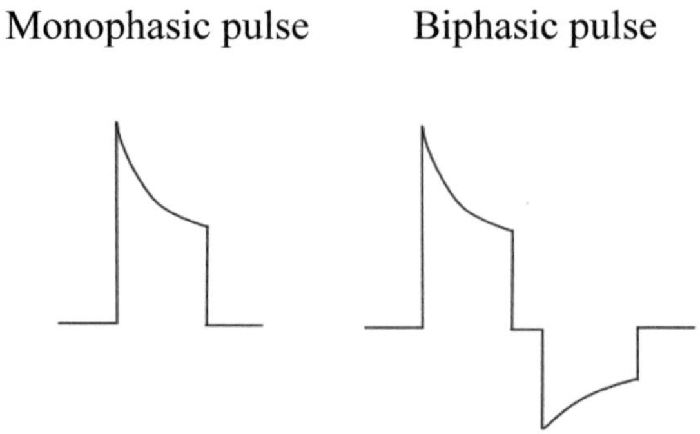

Monophasic pulse   Biphasic pulse

FIGURE 3.2 Left: monophasic pulse used during VF induction with T wave shock. Right: biphasic defibrillation pulse.

Pathway and Polarity

Another way to change the characteristics of the defibrillation pulse is to change the electrode starting as anode during pulse delivery. This feature has been given various names by different manufacturers—for example, pathway (Medtronic) or RV polarity (St. Jude Medical). It has, however, been difficult to show that a change in this parameter has a significant effect on DFT. The most common programming is to start the RV coil as the negative electrode (cathode) and to change this setting for one or two of the last therapies.

VF Therapies							
* SVC Coil Off		Rx1	Rx2	Rx3	Rx4	Rx5	Rx6
VF Therapy Status		On	On	On	On	On	On
Energy		35 J	35 J	35 J	35 J	35 J	35 J
Pathway		B>AX*	B>AX*	B>AX*	B>AX*	AX>B*	AX>B*
ATP...	Before Charging						

FIGURE 3.3 Example of a programming screen from a Medtronic Protecta. Programming of pathway is done either as B>AX (RV coil to Active can/SVC, where RV coil starts as cathode), or as AX>B (Active can/SVC to RV coil where Active can/SVC starts as cathode).

Different ICD Systems

The choice of ICD system is based on the indication for treatment and includes, for example:

- Possible brady arrhythmia with the need for pacemaker treatment
- Existing heart failure and the need for biventricular pacing (CRT)
- The need for specific features to detect and treat tachy arrhythmia, including atrial arrhythmias

Whether to use a single-chamber or a dual-chamber system mostly depends on the need for bradycardia stimulation and the wish for more advanced SVT discrimination. For selected patients, anti-tachy stimulation (ATP) may be indicated to convert certain types of atrial tachycardia. For atrial ATP therapy, a dual-chamber system is needed. Triple-chamber systems are chosen for patients indicated for biventricular CRT stimulation.

The ICD Lead

In early ICD systems, the defibrillation leads were placed directly on the heart, epicardially, during open heart surgery as so-called patches. Hence, this was a more complex procedure demanding thoracotomy. Modern ICDs use leads that are placed transvenously during a procedure much like a common pacemaker implantation.

An ICD lead is built much like a pacemaker lead, with the exception of one or two coils for high-power therapy. These coils are wound outside the outer insulation to allow for high-voltage delivery. The total area of a high-voltage electrode needs to be large in order not to cause myocardial burn, and the coil design combines a large area with a flexible lead body. In addition to one or two high-voltage coils, the lead also includes electrodes for sensing and pacing. Pacing and sensing configuration is usually strictly bipolar (lead tip to a ring approximately 10 mm from the tip), but some manufacturers use a so-called integrated configuration. For these systems, the lead tip and the high-voltage coil in the right ventricle (RV coil) are used for sensing and pacing.

RV Coil

All ICD leads are fit with a high-voltage lead in the right ventricle. This lead is referred to as the RV coil. Leads only equipped with *one* high-voltage electrode are called single-coil leads. Energy is then delivered between the RV coil and the can of the ICD. For successful defibrillation, an apical lead placement is preferred in order for the RV coil to cover as much of the left ventricular myocardium as possible during energy delivery. The electrical area of the RV coil is typically around 600 mm^2.

SVC Coil

The ICD lead may also be equipped with a second high-voltage electrode placed in the superior vena cava, a so-called SVC coil. This type of lead is called dual-coil and delivers energy between the RV coil and a combination of the SVC coil and can (electrically connected). Advantages of using a dual-coil lead may be:

- The larger electrode area creates lower electrical impedance, which allows for a faster and more effective energy delivery.
- A larger portion of the ventricular myocardium is covered during energy delivery, which increases the chances of successful defibrillation.

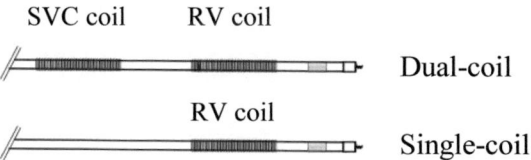

FIGURE 3.4 Top: dual-coil lead with SVC and RV coils on the same lead body. Bottom: single-coil lead with only an RV coil for defibrillation.

Since defibrillation threshold is difficult to measure, no clear evidence of better success rates for dual-coil versus single-coil exists. Dual-coil systems offer the possibility to use the SVC coil to register extracardiac EGM signals (between SVC coil and can), called leadless ECG. The signals registered are surface-ECG-like and make external ECG registration redundant. Leadless ECG is also an advantage when following patients remotely as well as during interpretation of stored EGM during arrhythmia, since morphology changes are more clearly visible than for the bipolar registration. Wide-QRS arrhythmias are more easily differentiated from arrhythmias with narrow QRS.

A few words on the possible disadvantage of using an SVC coil should also be mentioned. The primary concern is the body's ability to encapsulate the leads which is a more common problem if an SVC coil is used, due to the position of the coil against the wall of the vessel. Dual-coil leads may be more difficult to extract, should it be needed. However, modern leads use a silicone backfill in the coil to prevent tissue from penetrating between coil windings, which has significantly decreased this problem.

In contrast with what is described above, some patients exhibit a *higher* DFT with a dual-coil than with a single-coil configuration. This behavior is due to the fact that the energy density on the surface of the lead becomes higher if only one coil is used. In some patients, this is not balanced out by the higher coverage of ventricular tissue, and thus DFT increases when an SVC coil is active. There is some evidence that dual-coil might lead to lower DFT than single-coil, especially for patients with high DFT.[3]

In some modern devices, it is possible to noninvasively program the SVC coil to be active or inactive. However, this function is still missing in many systems, which means that a reoperation is necessary if the SVC coil needs to be deactivated.

---

[3] J Am Coll Cardiol 1998;31:1391-4

Various Connector Standards

Similar to the connector standard that exists for pacemakers, the IS-1, which guarantees mechanical compatibility between leads and pacemakers from different manufacturers, there are existing standards for high-voltage leads. The connector header for the ICD includes connectors for different types of leads. Presently there are two different standards for high-voltage lead connectors: DF-1 and DF-4. DF-4 was created more recently to allow for smaller connector headers, thereby decreasing the overall size of the device. For devices with a DF-1 connector, the connector standard IS-1 is used for the sense/pace connector.

DF-1

DF-1 was the first standard for defibrillation leads. The technology is built around a bifurcated or trifurcated lead connector, meaning that the lead body has two or three connectors to be connected into the ICD. When comparing DF-1 to IS-1, the IS-1 pin is thicker to prevent a pacemaker IS-1) lead from being connected to a high-voltage DF-1 port. If this was to happen, and defibrillation therapy was to be delivered on the small-surfaced pacemaker electrodes, serious burn of the cardiac tissue would result. The high energy, together with the small area, would create a situation very much like an ablation procedure. Similar to the IS-1, the DF-1 standard places the sealing rings on the lead connector. DF-1 connectors are unipolar.

DF-4

A new standard for defibrillation lead connectors was launched in 2010. With the increasing number of CRT-D implants, which include an additional left ventricular (LV) lead, the connector header was causing devices to be large and bulky. To decrease the overall volume, a more streamlined connector was needed, preferably with only one connection to the ICD. The solution was an inline connector which is either tripolar (bipolar sense/pace and unipolar high-voltage) or quadripolar (with the addition of an extra unipolar, high-voltage SVC lead). In contrast to DF-1 and IS-1, DF-4 has the sealing rings inside the ICD port.

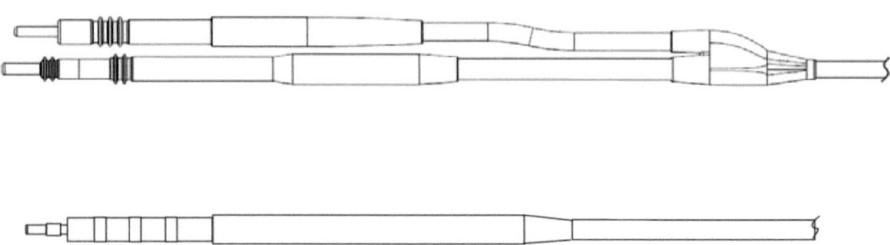

FIGURE 3.5 Different connector standards for ICD leads. Top: DF-1/IS-1 connector. Bottom: DF-4 connector.

Placement of the Ports

Different manufacturers use different placement of the connector ports in the ICD header. This is unfortunate since it is of utmost importance that connections between the lead and the ICD are correct, both for connecting the right lead to the right port and for the connection itself.

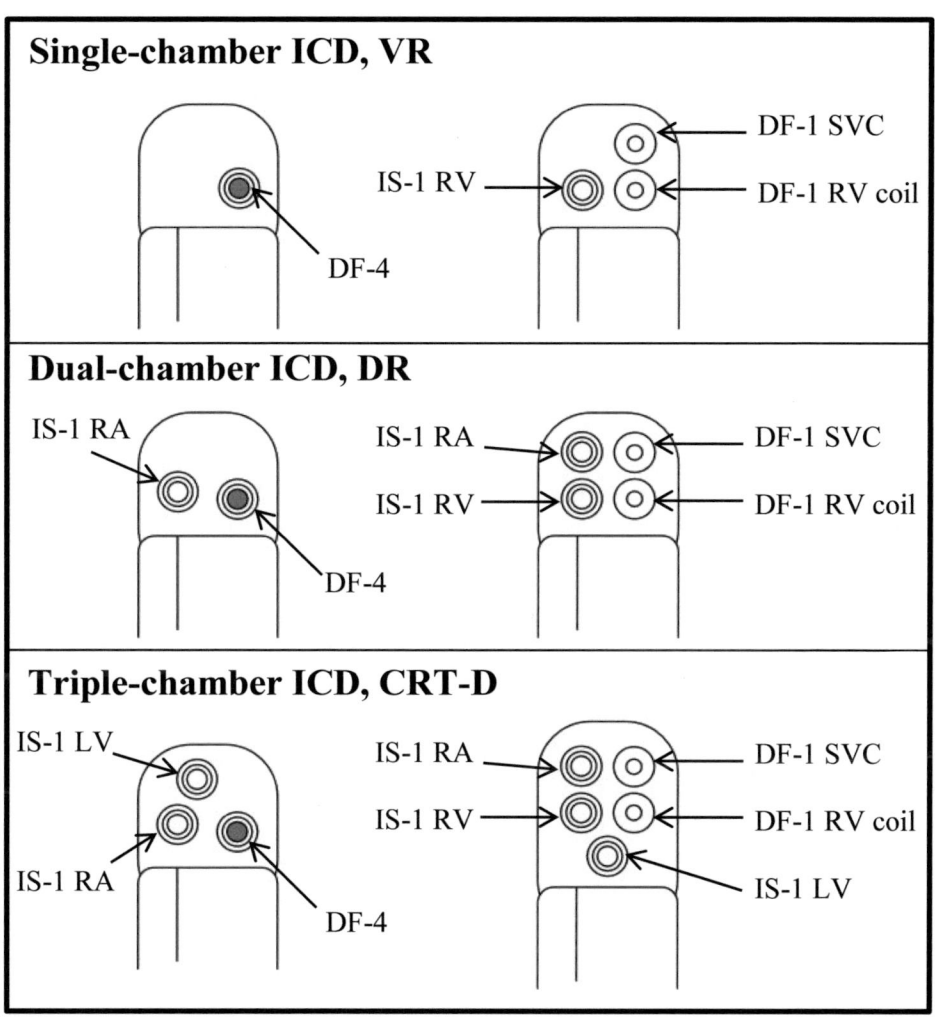

FIGURE 2.6 Example of connector ports (Medtronic) with different connector standards. Left: DF-4. Right: DF-1.

The Single-Chamber System

In addition to the ICD itself, the single-chamber system consists of an ICD lead placed in the right ventricular apex. This lead may be of a single-coil or a dual-coil type and has bipolar or integrated pacing polarity. The single-chamber ICD may be programmed to VVI or VVIR mode and allows for anti-tachy therapies (ATP), defibrillation, and cardioversion of the ventricles.

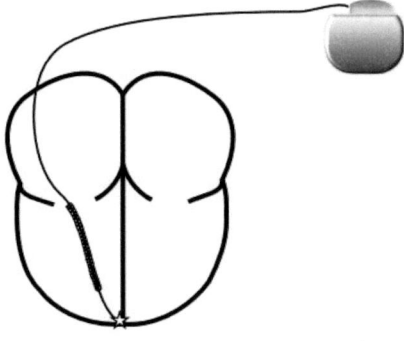

FIGURE 3.7 Single-chamber system with one lead, placed in the right ventricle.

The Dual-Chamber System

In addition to what is found in the single-chamber system, the dual-chamber system also has a pacemaker lead placed in the right atrium. This allows for sensing and stimulation of the atrium in so-called DDD or DDDR mode. Some ICDs have the ability to deliver therapies in the atrium as well (for example, ATP). An ICD with an atrial sensing lead also has a better chance of differentiating between true VT/VF and SVT since information about the atrial rate may be compared to that of the ventricle.

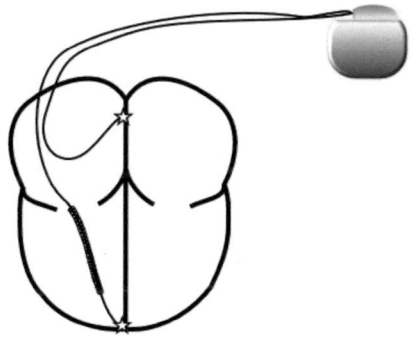

FIGURE 3.8 Dual-chamber system with one lead placed in the right ventricle and one in the right atrium.

The Triple-Chamber System

The triple-chamber system, or CRT-D system, is used in patients indicated for biventricular heart failure pacing in addition to ICD therapy. The system uses an ICD lead (single-coil or dual-coil) placed in the right ventricular apex, a pacing lead placed in the right atrium, and a left ventricular lead (LV lead) placed in the coronary sinus. Hence, this system adds biventricular pacing to the dual-chamber ICD described above.

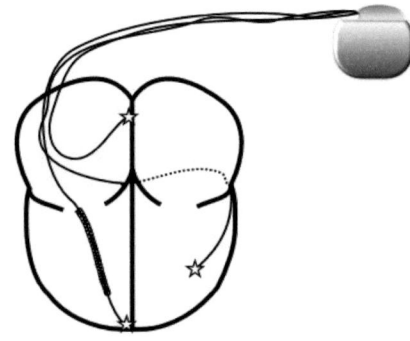

FIGURE 3.9 Triple-chamber system with one lead in the right ventricle, one in the right atrium, and one outside of the left ventricle in the coronary sinus.

Indications and Guidelines

ICD treatment is a comparatively new therapy still under development. The first ICD, developed by Polish physician Michel Mirowski, was implanted in Baltimore, Maryland, in 1980. Development started to take off in the second half of the 1990s, and ICD guidelines have been updated on several occasions as new study results have expanded the indications to larger patient populations. Distinction is made between primary and secondary prevention therapies, where primary prevention therapy has increased substantially over the last years.

Clinical Evidence

There is strong clinical evidence that ICD treatment may decrease mortality in selected patient populations. The treatment is also cost effective from a health economics perspective. Nevertheless, only some patients indicated for an ICD will get one, even though the U.S. is better off than most other Western countries.

Some of the more important studies on which current guidelines are based are briefly summarized below.

MADIT-II

The MADIT-II study,[4] published in the New England Journal of Medicine in March 2002, included 1232 patients after myocardial infarction with an EF ≤ 30%. The patients were randomized 3:2 to ICD or conventional pharmaceutical treatment. The primary endpoint was death from any cause. In November 2001, the study was prematurely stopped. The reason was an interim analysis showing that the patients in the ICD arm had a 31% mortality reduction compared to the patients in the control arm. In July 2002, the FDA approved primary prevention ICD treatment based on MADIT-II indications.

DEFINITE

The DEFIbrillators in Non-Ischemic cardiomyopathy Treatment Evaluation[5] was published in NEJM in 2004. The study included 458 patients with non-ischemic dilated cardiomyopathy, EF < 36%, and frequent PVCs or non-sustained VT, randomized to optimal medical therapy (OMT) or OMT plus ICD. The primary endpoint was death from any cause, and the secondary endpoint was death caused by arrhythmia. Fewer patients died in the ICD arm (primary endpoint: death from any cause), but the result was only statistically borderline significant (p = 0.08). However, for patients in NYHA class III, a significant reduction of death from any cause was seen. ICD treatment significantly reduced the risk of sudden death caused by arrhythmia in this patient population.

---

[4] N Engl J Med 2002;346:877-83
[5] N Engl J Med 2004;350:2151-8

DINAMIT

Several studies undertaken before DINAMIT[6] (the Defibrillator IN Acute Myocardial Infarction Trial) had shown that ICD treatment could reduce mortality in patients with heart disease and an increased risk for ventricular arrhythmias. However, there were insufficient larger studies showing the benefit for patients early after myocardial infarction (MI). The DINAMIT study included patients with reduced LVEF ($\leq 35\%$) and impaired cardiac autonomic function (depressed heart-rate variability or an elevated average 24-hour heart-rate on Holter monitoring), 6 to 40 days after MI. The primary outcome was death from any cause. Death from arrhythmia was the predefined secondary outcome. The outcome of the study was somewhat unexpected. Although the ICD group had significantly lower mortality caused by arrhythmias (-58%), this was balanced out by an increased mortality in non-arrhythmic deaths, compared to the control group. There was no difference in the primary endpoint between the two groups. The conclusion, therefore, is that ICD treatment early after myocardial infarction (< 40 days) is not recommended. DINAMIT was published in the New England Journal of Medicine in 2004.

SCD-HeFT

The Sudden Cardiac Death in Heart Failure Trial[7] studied heart failure patients in NYHA class II–III with EF $< 35\%$. 2521 patients were randomized to one of three groups: placebo, Amiodarone, or ICD. The study was published in NEJM in 2005. Approximately half of the patients suffered from ischemic heart failure. Although no difference in mortality

---

[6] N Engl J Med 2004;351:2481-8
[7] N Engl J Med 2005;352:225-37

was found between the placebo and the Amiodarone groups, mortality was 23% lower for the ICD group—an absolute difference of 7.2%! Before SCD-HeFT, no published studies existed that showed that treatment with an ICD could decrease mortality for patients without previous cardiac arrest. There were also no studies showing the effect on patients with ischemic heart failure. With SCD-HeFT, clear evidence was found that ICD implant as primary preventive treatment decreases mortality for both ischemic and non-ischemic heart failure patients.

The NBG Code

In order to simplify the way we describe pacemaker and ICD basic functions, so-called NBG codes are used. This universal code system describes the pacemaker/ICD basic functions and gives information about the specific mode. NBG is short for NASPE/BPEG Generic Pacemaker Code, and is the result of a cooperation between the North American (NASPE, North American Society for Pacing and Electrophysiology) and the British (BPEG, British Pacing & Electrophysiology Group) societies for pacing and electrophysiology. Different codes exist for pacemakers and ICDs. The ICD code system is built upon four-letter combinations where every position (I–IV) has its own specific meaning.

- **Position I**: The first position indicates where in the heart the ICD may deliver defibrillation therapy. This can be in the atrium (A), in the ventricle (V), both in the atrium and in the ventricle (D = double), or not at all (O).

- **Position II**: The second position indicates in which heart chamber/chambers the ICD can deliver anti-tachycardia pacing (ATP). This also can be in the atrium (A), in the ventricle (V), both in the atrium and in the ventricle (D = double), or not at all (O).

- **Position III**: The third position indicates the way in which the ICD detects arrhythmia. When the NBG codes were developed, there was a general belief that detection in the future would be done either by sensing the electrical signals of the heart—i.e., the electrogram (E)—or by detecting hemodynamic differences by means of a hemodynamic sensor (H). Presently only the electrogram is used to differentiate between arrhythmia and normal sinus rhythm.

- **Position IV**: The fourth position indicates what type of pacemaker is included in the ICD, or more specifically, in which heart chamber/chambers bradycardia stimulation may be delivered. Similar to positions I and II, the different possibilities are in the atrium (A), in the ventricle (V), both in the atrium and in the ventricle (D = double), or not at all (O).

It is, however, not uncommon to use the pacemaker NBG codes to describe ICD function also, looking at the number of heart chambers treated:
- Single-chamber ICD, or VVI-ICD
- Dual-chamber ICD, or DDD-ICD
- Biventricular (triple-chamber) ICD, or CRT-D

Position	I	II	III	IV
	Heart chamber for defibrillation	**Heart chamber for ATP**	**Arrhythmia detection**	**Anti-bradycardia stimulation**
	O = None	**O** = None	**E** = Electrogram	**O** = None
	A = Atrium	**A** = Atrium	**H** = Hemodynamic	**A** = Atrium
	V = Ventricle	**V** = Ventricle		**V** = Ventricle
	D = Double (A+V)	**D** = Double (A+V)		**D** = Double

Table 4.1 The letter combinations of the NBG code for ICD

The Pacemaker System

The first ICD systems did not include pacemaker functions since their primary task was to save lives in patients who had survived ventricular fibrillation. Technology has since then moved forward in the field of ICDs, and more and more features have been added to the original "shock-box." Today's ICDs incorporate a modern single-chamber, dual-chamber, or biventricular (CRT) pacemaker. In the early history of ICD treatment, it was not uncommon for patients to receive not only an ICD but also an additional separate pacemaker! This was both unpractical and difficult to handle since the two systems could easily interact, with lethal results. Having a pacemaker integrated in the ICD system is therefore advantageous and is offered in all ICD systems today. It is not within the scope of this book to fully describe the functions of a pacemaker since this has already been done in the book *Pacemaker Programming—A Handbook*, by the same author, released in 2013.

The pacemaker part of the ICD mainly fulfills three different needs:

- Bradycardia protection for patients with sick sinus syndrome, AV block, etc.
- Bradycardia stimulation after treatment and termination of tachycardia, which may otherwise be followed by a shorter or longer asystole.
- Anti-tachycardia pacing to terminate atrial or ventricular tachycardia.

Sensing in the ICD

It is of utmost importance that sensing in the ICD works almost perfectly both in the atrium (if applicable) and in the ventricle. A correct sensing function may be even more important in an ICD than it is in a pacemaker because of the need to correctly detect the small electric signals during ventricular fibrillation without oversensing of, for example, T waves or extracardiac signals during sinus rhythm. The sensitivity is therefore higher in an ICD than in a pacemaker. A common setting for ventricular sensitivity is 0.3 mV (compared to 2.8–4 mV for a pacemaker). These high demands have led to the development of different sensing algorithms for ICDs than what are commonly used in pacemakers.

Auto-Adjusted Sensing

A pacemaker uses a fixed sensing level, meaning that a signal of a certain size will always trigger sensing independent of where in the heart cycle it appears. Unlike a pacemaker, an ICD uses auto-adjusted sensing, meaning that the sensitivity level changes with the phases of the heart cycle. Sensing is adjusted, from beat to beat, to a level adapted to the amplitude of the sensed signal. A signal that is large enough to be sensed during one moment of the heart cycle may still be too small to be sensed in another. The advantage of this algorithm is that it is possible to avoid, for example, oversensing of pathological T waves, while at the same time allowing for correct sensing of small fibrillation waves with even lower amplitudes.

Auto-adjusted sensing works similarly across all models, although the details may differ when looking more closely at the algorithms. In this book I have chosen to concentrate on the principles, referring readers interested in the smaller details to the individual product manuals.

The programmed sensitivity value in an ICD refers to the highest sensitivity level (lowest mV value) that can be reached during a heart cycle. However, during most of the heart cycle, the sensitivity is much lower (higher mV value). This is achieved by adjusting the sensitivity automatically on every sensed or paced event. As an example, a sensed R wave will lead to adjustment of the sensitivity level to approximately 75% of the sensed amplitude of the signal (this differs somewhat between models and may even be programmable in some). With this type of algorithm, an R wave of 12 mV would lead to a sensitivity of 9 mV for a short period of time. However, the algorithm often has some sort of limitation as to how insensitive it is allowed to be. In a Medtronic ICD, for example, the value is limited to 10 times the programmed sensitivity, which, at the standard programming of 0.3 mV, will lead to a maximum value of 3 mV. The sensitivity value (in mV) then slowly falls until the programmed value is reached or another R wave is detected. In some systems, it is possible to program the so-called decay delay, allowing the sensitivity value to stay at the higher value (lower sensitivity) during a programmable time before the decrement down to the programmed value is initiated.

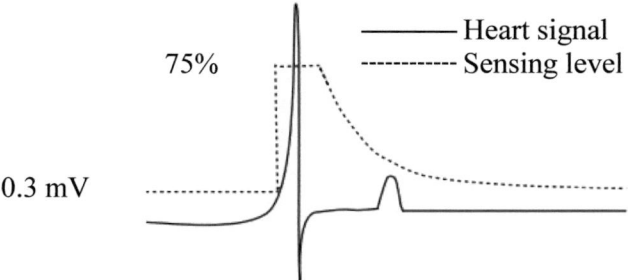

FIGURE 5.1 Auto-adjusted sensing. When the amplitude of the EGM signal exceeds the programmed sensitivity (in this example 0.3 mV), the sensitivity decreases to 75% of the measured signal amplitude. After the blanking period (or after the programmed decay delay), the sensitivity is increased following a predefined curve until the programmed sensitivity has been reached or another signal is detected.

Some of the more commonly seen ICD sensing problems are T wave oversensing (in the ventricular channel) and sensing of far-field R waves (FFRW) in the atrial channel. They will both lead to double-counting of the signals during the heart cycle, which may have consequences in the way the ICD detects arrhythmia. Since both T wave and FFRW oversensing arise early after the sensed R wave/P wave, this type of problem often may be solved through the auto-adjusted sensing algorithm. The ICD is relatively insensitive directly after the sensed signal, thereby leaving the unwanted signal (T wave or FFRW) below the sensing level.

Oversensing

T Wave Oversensing

For the ICD to be able to sense a signal, the signal not only needs to exceed the sensing level in amplitude but also needs to have the right frequency content to pass the ICD input filter. This filter is adapted to filter out signals of different frequency content than those of the R wave and the P wave. A normal T wave usually does not fully pass the filter (frequency content too low), causing the resulting amplitude after the filter to be low. However, in some patients with more pathological T waves, the T wave has a higher amplitude with a more pointed morphology, and thus also has a higher frequency content. This may be enough to let a larger part of the T wave pass the filter, leading to filtered amplitudes high enough to be sensed.

Sensing of the T wave may have various causes and is most problematic when heart rate is high. Since continuous T wave oversensing is perceived by the ICD as double the heart rate, the phenomenon may result in therapy being delivered at heart rates of half the lowest rate programmed for detection.

A common reason for T wave oversensing is ischemia during exercise, leading to changes in T wave morphology and frequency content. The T wave is then sensed as the heart rate increases, which may lead to inappropriate therapy. The phenomenon may be difficult to provoke, which makes it difficult to prove that efforts to solve the problem have been successful.

However, the most common reason for T wave oversensing is diminishing R waves. When the R wave amplitude approaches that of the T wave, auto-adjusted sensitivity may not succeed in differentiating the two, leading to sensing of both R wave and T wave. Success of the algorithm is dependent on the R wave being sufficiently larger that the T wave in order to generate a sensing level (75% of R wave amplitude) that exceeds the T wave amplitude. When the R wave is small and the T wave large in amplitude, T wave oversensing is more likely to happen. This can prove very difficult to solve by programming alone (in some cases, a change to integrated sensing polarity may solve the problem), and often calls for repositioning the RV lead or adding a separate sense/pace lead. In some newer devices, a special algorithm that differentiates the T wave from the R wave is available so as to avoid inappropriate therapy based on T wave oversensing (for example, the Medtronic TWOS algorithm).

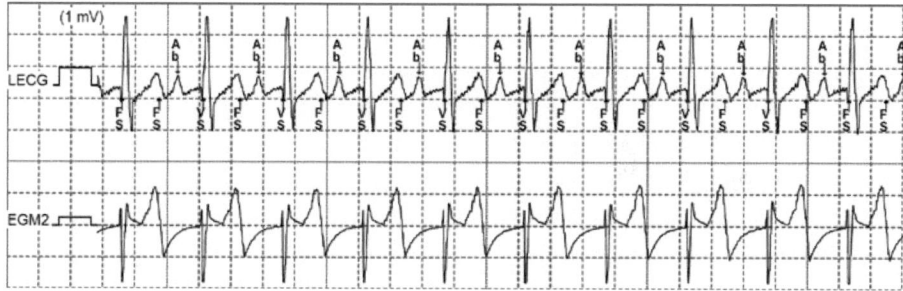

FIGURE 5.2 Example of T wave oversensing. Top: EGM registration with an extracardiac registration (leadless ECG). Bottom: a bipolar ventricular EGM. Note the large T waves on the lower registration, together with the ICD markers varying between VS (ventricular sense below the VT zone) and FS (fast sense in the VF zone). If this pattern is sustained at a slightly higher rate, the ICD may detect VF and deliver VF therapy.

FFRW Sensing

When the ICD is sensing cardiac activity, it is important that only signals from the heart chamber where the lead is placed be sensed. However, it may happen that the atrial lead also detects the R wave signal from the ventricle. This signal, so-called far-field R wave (FFRW), consists of the summed signal from the ventricles registered by the atrial lead, similar to an ECG. FFRW signals may often be differentiated from the intracardiac P waves by their lower frequency content as well as their commonly smaller amplitude. A FFRW is reminiscent of a surface ECG signal with broader morphology than the intracardiac signals. Double-sensing in the atrial channel may lead to the ICD concluding that the rhythm is an atrial arrhythmia with 2:1 conduction, which can lead to mode-switching if mode-switch is activated.

P Wave Oversensing

When programmed for integrated sensing polarity, the ICD measures the difference in potential between the RV tip and RV coil. For this to work safely, it is important that the RV coil not protrude into the atrium. If the coil is too long or not placed apically enough, P waves may be sensed on the ventricular channel, possibly leading to detection and inappropriate therapy.

Non-Physiologic Oversensing

Even in bipolar sensing configuration, oversensing of extracardiac signals may sometimes occur. This is a serious occurrence since the ICD may interpret the signals as VF if sustained. The worst cases of sensing of external signals often involve water as a component. This could be a faulty electric floor-heating system in the shower, leaking current in therapeutic baths, etc. These kinds of problems are difficult to protect against and may not be easily solved by programming. It is important to look through all stored episodes during follow-up, even when the patient didn't receive therapy. Episodes terminated before therapy was delivered are stored as non-sustained VT (NS-VT). External noise most often has very short VV intervals and can typically be seen simultaneously in more than one lead or sensing configuration. If noise has been detected and stored as arrhythmia, it is important to investigate where the patient was when the noise was detected, and continue the investigation from there. Never let the patient leave the clinic without doing everything possible to make sure that this will not happen again.

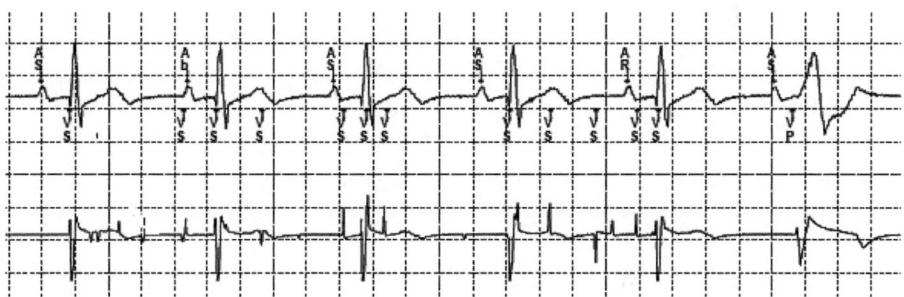

FIGURE 5.3 Oversensing of noise from a fractured sense/pace lead. Note the extra markers and the small signal spikes between R waves on the lower EGM tracing.

Undersensing

There are three different types of undersensing in ICDs:
- Undersensing of R waves
- Undersensing of P waves
- Undersensing during arrhythmia

Each type of undersensing has different consequences.

R Wave Undersensing

R wave undersensing during sinus rhythm may lead to pacemaker stimulation in the ventricle, even though it is not necessary. This is extremely uncommon due to the high sensitivity (commonly 0.3 mV) used by the ICD. If the ICD is not able to detect ventricular signals, stimulation pulses will be delivered asynchronously in the heart cycle and possibly induce arrhythmias.

Even though undersensing of the R wave is extremely uncommon, it sometimes happens that the R wave amplitude decreases with time, or shortly after implantation. This is worrying in more ways than one. When the R wave is small, there may be reason to suspect that amplitudes during an eventual arrhythmia (mostly VF) are even smaller. If so, the ICD may not detect VF, leading to no delivered therapy. Also, the risk for T wave oversensing increases with smaller R wave amplitudes.

Undersensing of the P Wave

Undersensing the P wave will normally not lead to significant problems as long as the ventricular rate doesn't fall into any of the detection zones. If discriminators against atrial arrhythmias based on AV analysis are used, these may incorrectly conclude that the atrial rate is lower than the ventricular rate, thereby misinterpreting the rhythm. If the ventricular rate found in the detection zone is higher than that of the atria, the ICD will interpret the rhythm as VT/VF and deliver therapy if the rhythm is sustained. It is therefore important that atrial sensing be functioning correctly to ensure correct ICD function.

Blanking Period and Refractory Period

As described above, it is of utmost importance that the ICD correctly senses all heart signals, and at the same time avoids sensing any other signals such as T waves, external noise, etc. To accomplish optimal sensing, a combination of programmed values for sensitivity, blanking periods, and refractory periods is used. The blanking period is a short time period following every sensed signal, stimulation pulse, or high-voltage shock. During this period, no sensing can take place. The refractory period takes over after the end of the blanking period, or to be more specific, the programmed refractory period starts with the blanking period. During the refractory period, sensing is possible but is registered as refractory sensing and thus is not allowed to affect ICD timing. Refractory sensed events are ignored by the ICD's pacemaker functions but are used for arrhythmia detection.

Blanking Periods

In the dual-chamber ICD, eight (8) different blanking periods exist. Usually they are not all programmable. It is important to note that the various companies use different terminologies. In some companies (e.g., Medtronic and Boston Scientific) the time period when the ICD is "blind" to any signals is called the blanking period, while in other companies (e.g., St. Jude Medical) it is called the refractory period (absolute and relative). In this book I have chosen to use the term "blanking period" for the time period when the ICD is unable to sense, and "refractory period" for the time period when sensing is possible but does not affect ICD timing.

The atrial blanking period starts after atrial sensing, atrial stimulation, and ventricular stimulation.

The ventricular blanking period starts after ventricular sensing, ventricular stimulation, and atrial stimulation.

The blanking period after stimulation is programmed to be longer than that after sensing in order to minimize the risk of sensing the atrial or ventricular polarization signals as well.

Blanking periods that are started in the *opposite chamber* after stimulation are called cross-chamber blanking and prevent far-field sensing of the stimulation pulse in the opposite chamber (crosstalk).

Blanking periods are also started in each channel after high-voltage shock. However, this blanking period is not programmable and is commonly in the range of 500 ms.

To give an idea about the length of the different blanking periods, the table below illustrates common programmed values. Please note that changes to these values may be needed for the individual patient.

Parameter	Blanking period (ms)
Atrial blanking after atrial stimulation	200
Atrial blanking after atrial sensing	100
Atrial blanking after ventricular stimulation	30
Ventricular blanking after ventricular stimulation	200
Ventricular blanking after ventricular sensing	120
Ventricular blanking after atrial stimulation	30
Ventricular blanking after high-voltage therapy	520
Atrial blanking after high-voltage therapy	520

Table 5.1 The different blanking periods in the ICD.

Refractory Periods

PVARP (Post Ventricular Atrial Refractory Period) and PVAB (Post Ventricular Atrial Blanking) is started in the ICD in the same way as in a pacemaker, i.e., in the atrium after a ventricular event. In the ICD, these parameters are only used for the pacemaker part of the device, and also signals sensed in the PVARP are used for arrhythmia detection.

Polarity

Bipolar Polarity

The sensing polarity in the ICD is most commonly bipolar. To be able to sense, or stimulate, two electrical poles are necessary. During stimulation, current travels from one pole to the other, and during sensing, the difference in voltage potential between the poles is measured. The tip of the lead always constitutes one pole, while the other pole is either a ring placed proximally on the lead in the heart (bipolar sensing) or is represented by the RV coil (integrated sensing). Unipolar sensing is not allowed in the ICD (lead tip to can). Although it has the advantage of being vector independent, the high sensitivity levels (low mV values) in the ICD would make the unipolar system too prone to oversensing. Unipolar sensing polarity in an ICD would radically increase the risk for oversensing and, with it, the risk for inappropriate high-voltage therapies.

Bipolar stimulation and sensing polarities are the most common in ICDs today. This makes the system relatively insensitive to external noise, even if it sometimes proves non-optimal for sensing R waves with disadvantageous vector spread.

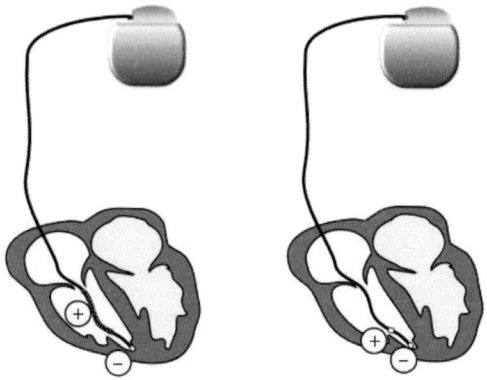

FIGURE 5.4 Pacing and sensing polarity. Left: integrated polarity with the RV coil as anode and the RV tip as cathode. Right: bipolar polarity with RV ring as anode and RV tip as cathode.

Integrated Sensing

Integrated polarity is more common for some manufacturers (e.g., Boston Scientific), and is defined by sensing and pacing between RV tip and RV coil. This type of system is slightly more sensitive to external noise, but on the other hand, it is less sensitive to vector spread. In some modern systems, it is possible to choose between bipolar and integrated polarity, given a suitable lead has been implanted.

Adding a Separate Pace/Sense Lead

At times, the goal to place the RV lead in an apical position for best coverage of the ventricular myocardium, while at the same time finding optimal sensing and stimulation thresholds, may prove difficult to achieve. In such a situation, it is possible to abandon the low-voltage part of the ICD lead and instead place a separate pace/sense (pacemaker) lead higher up on the septal wall, for example. This may also be a solution for patients with T wave oversensing. Note that this practice is sparsely used in the U.S, to keep the number of implanted leads at a minimum, but may be of help in specific patients.

Lower Rate

Lower rate in an ICD is the same as lower rate in a pacemaker. The delivered stimulation rate depends on the programmed lower rate but also on the programmed mode.

VVI: When the intrinsic rate falls below the lower rate, the ICD stimulates the ventricle at the programmed lower rate.

DDD: When the intrinsic rate falls below the lower rate, the ICD stimulates the atrium at the programmed lower rate. If no ventricular event is sensed before the end of the AV interval, the ventricle is stimulated. During sensed atrial activity above the lower rate but below the upper rate, the ventricle is stimulated, if needed, at the end of the AV interval. In this way, rate variation is achieved by following the sinus node.

While lower rate may be critical for a pacemaker patient, ICD patients often don't have the need for bradycardia stimulation. Only about 10% of ICD patients also have an indication for pacing (although the number is higher if counting the patients with need for stimulation due to asystole immediately after arrhythmia termination). It is therefore not uncommon to program the ICD to VVI with a lower rate of 30 bpm. This programming minimizes unnecessary ventricular stimulation but allows for bradycardia/asystole protection.

For ICD patients with a parallel indication for bradycardia pacing, lower rate is programmed in the same way as for a pacemaker patient, commonly 60–70 bpm.

Amplitude and Pulse Width

Programming of amplitude and pulse width is done much in the same way as for a pacemaker patient, meaning that the threshold is measured for the implanted leads, and programmed values are set according to measurement results. A safety margin of two times the amplitude, or possibly three times the pulse width, is common. However, in the ICD there is a difference between the output of the pulses for bradycardia stimulation and those used for ATP therapy or stimulation after high-voltage therapy. The latter are normally programmed to higher amplitude, and possibly also pulse width, to secure capture even during fast arrhythmias that sometimes lead to increased threshold values.

The Technical Construction of the ICD System

ICD Battery

Demands on ICD batteries are a bit different from those on a pacemaker battery. Above all, it is the need to drain a high amount of current out of the battery in a short time that differs between the two applications. To facilitate a higher current drain, the ICD battery uses a different chemistry than that of the pacemaker battery. The positive pole (anode), however, is the same: lithium. The negative pole (cathode) in the pacemaker battery is usually iodine, while the cathode in the ICD battery more commonly consists of silver and vanadium oxide. While pacemaker battery voltage at beginning of service (BOS, the point in time when the battery is connected to the device electronics) is approximately 2.8 V, the ICD voltage is somewhat higher, 3.0–3.2 V depending on battery model. The lithium-silver-vanadium-oxide battery also has a higher energy density, meaning that the physical size of the battery can be kept small in spite of the large energy capacity. Battery capacity at BOS is commonly around 1 Ah (Ampere hour).

Longevity

The remaining longevity of an ICD is somewhat more difficult to project than that of a pacemaker. This is due to its ability to deliver high energy treatment. Factors affecting total longevity are mainly the following:

- Battery capacity
- Internal current drain, i.e., the current needed to keep the ICD electronics alive
- Amount of brady-stimulation and the lower rate
- Programmed amplitude and pulse width
- Amount of delivered ATP therapy sequences
- Lead impedance of the leads used for stimulation
- Number of high-voltage capacitor charges (formation as well as high-voltage therapy)

In a pacemaker, the mean current drain is often more or less stable over time, which is not necessarily true for an ICD. For example, an electrical storm may lead to delivery of multiple high-voltage shocks, thereby draining the battery in a short time. Also, the ICD battery with its different chemistry often has a less linear discharge curve than that of a pacemaker. It is not uncommon for these types of batteries to have a plateau somewhere on the discharge curve, which makes predictions of remaining longevity even more difficult, especially if battery voltage and impedance are used as indicators.

When making sure that a system with a long longevity is chosen, it is not enough to just look at the battery capacity, or even calculated longevity at 100% stimulation. Specially designed algorithms to minimize unnecessary ventricular stimulation may increase longevity, as well as algorithms for automatic measurement and adjustment of amplitude and pulse width.

High-Voltage Capacitors

As described above, an ICD battery has a battery voltage of approximately 3.2 V, and a defibrillation pulse is delivered at approximately 750–800 V! This may seem like an impossible equation, but it is achieved by the use of high-voltage capacitors. A capacitor is an electronic component used to store electrical energy. When the capacitor is charged, the energy can be delivered in a very short time, in this case as a defibrillation pulse to the heart. Current is drained from the battery to charge the capacitors to the desired energy over a number of seconds and is thereafter delivered to the heart during a few milliseconds.

Charge Time

Once the ICD detects a life-threatening arrhythmia, it is important that therapy be delivered as soon as possible. The probability of converting VF decreases with the time the heart has been in VF. The more time that passes, the more difficult to terminate the arrhythmia. The time it takes to charge the capacitors may therefore play an important role in whether the therapy is going to be effective or not. Various factors affect the charge time:

- Battery type and condition, i.e., how much energy has already been used. A new battery has lower internal impedance and can therefore deliver current more quickly than a more discharged one. The difference between a new and an old battery depends on battery technology. Some models have large differences, while the degree of discharge may only marginally affect the charge time in other models.
- Capacitor design and condition. The ability to charge quickly depends on the capacitor used but also, in some models, depends on when the

capacitor was last charged. A capacitor that hasn't been used for a long time has a higher resistance to charging and thus a longer charge time. To keep charge time to a minimum, the capacitors are automatically charged at regular time intervals, even when no energy needs to be delivered to the heart. This is done by the ICD parameter capacitor formation (Medtronic), maintenance charge (St. Jude Medical), or capacitor re-form (Boston Scientific). Technology is also moving forward in the field of capacitors, and new models that do not need to be reformed (thereby also saving some energy) are already on the market.

Capacitor charge time should ideally not exceed 10 seconds, even shorter if possible. This is an area where manufacturers may differ, with some systems allowing for up to 30 seconds before alerting due to long charge time. It is important to remember that charge time is always a delay of therapy. Most ICDs have a built-in warning system that will trigger an alarm if charge time becomes too long, since this can adversely affect therapy success. Please note that a *desired* delay of therapy to give time for the arrhythmia to self-terminate is programmed in the parameter NID (number of intervals to detect) or duration.

Capacitor Formation

Regular charging of the capacitors keeps charge times short, but also drains battery current corresponding to delivery of a full energy shock. This will adversely affect battery longevity (a little less than one month longevity is used for every charge), so it is important to optimize the time interval between capacitor formations.

To keep charge times short, the ICD will charge its capacitors regularly as described above. For such a formation to be as effective as possible—i.e., to shorten the charge time as much as possible—the energy should be left in the capacitor. The energy then slowly "leaks" out of the capacitor and is completely gone after approximately ten minutes. Since this is not the case when therapy is delivered in a high-voltage shock, formations are performed also if therapy has been delivered. The frequency with which capacitor formations take place differs between manufacturers and is usually programmable. For most devices, this is done every three to six months. Some manufacturers offer the ability to let the ICD decide when the next formation should take place based on, for example, delivered high-voltage therapy. As an example, a Medtronic ICD postpones the next automatic formation by 27 days if defibrillation therapy has been delivered. This prolongs longevity while keeping charge time to a minimum. With the use of newer capacitors which do not need reformation, ICD longevity may be increased by up to a year without other changes.

Detection

Whether an ICD will judge a rhythm as normal (sinus rhythm), or as an arrhythmia that needs to be treated, depends on the programming of the detection parameters. The decision is based on sensing of the EGM signals from the ventricle and, in dual-chamber devices, from the atrium. For an arrhythmia to be detected, the sensed signals need to be above a certain programmed rate (in a so-called detection zone) and be sustained. Different counters monitor the number of beats found within the detection zone, and at a programmed number of beats (Medtronic, St. Jude Medical) or after a preprogrammed time (Boston Scientific), arrhythmia is detected. To differentiate between supraventricular and ventricular arrhythmias, discriminator algorithms are used. These algorithms do not only take into account ventricular rate when evaluating rhythm and thus may decrease the risk of inappropriate therapies. If a fast ventricular rhythm is determined to be the result of atrial tachycardia, therapy will not be delivered. If the patient suffers a tachyarrhythmia within the rate zone for detection, the ICD will react in three steps:

1 Detection of the arrhythmia: the ICD decides whether and what type of therapy should be delivered
2 Therapy delivery: depending on which zone the arrhythmia is found in, and what therapies are programmed for that zone, the ICD delivers therapy to terminate the arrhythmia.

3   Evaluate the success of the delivered therapy (re-detection or termination): after therapy is delivered, the ICD continues to monitor heart rhythm to see whether the therapy was successful (termination) or whether the arrhythmia is still ongoing (re-detection). If the arrhythmia is re-detected, the ICD will continue to the next therapy for the given detection zone.

Detection Zones

Whether or not a rhythm is interpreted as arrhythmia depends on the rates programmed for the detection zone or zones (up to three zones may be programmed). These zones define at what ventricular rates arrhythmia should be detected and are commonly called VF (ventricular fibrillation) and VT (ventricular tachycardia) zones. By activating more than one zone, different therapies may be delivered depending on the rate of the arrhythmia. One set of therapies may be programmed for arrhythmias with rates falling within the VT zone and another set for arrhythmias within the VF zone. When two zones are activated, both a lower rate limit and an upper rate limit are defined. Rates above the lower rate limit for the VT zone, but below the lower rate limit for VF, are interpreted as VT and treated with VT therapy if sustained. Rates above the lower rate limit for VF lead to VF therapy if sustained.

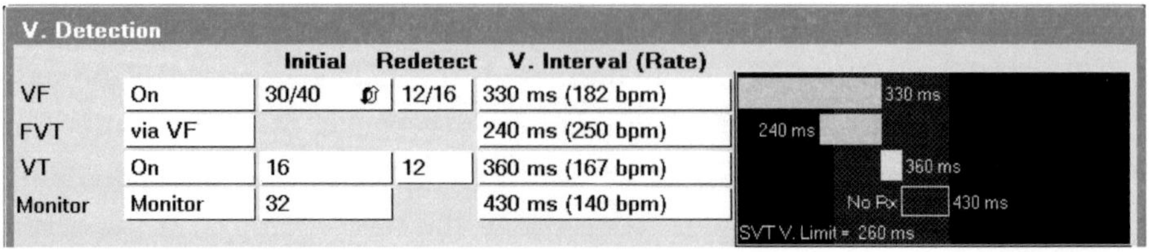

V. Detection		Initial	Redetect	V. Interval (Rate)	
VF	On	30/40	12/16	330 ms (182 bpm)	330 ms
FVT	via VF			240 ms (250 bpm)	240 ms
VT	On	16	12	360 ms (167 bpm)	360 ms
Monitor	Monitor	32		430 ms (140 bpm)	No Rx 430 ms
					SVT V. Limit = 260 ms

FIGURE 7.1 Programmer screen from a Medtronic Protecta. Note the way the rate limits are shown: 140–167 bpm represent the monitor zone (without therapies), 167–182 bpm represent the VT zone, 182–250 bpm represent the FVT zone, and rates above 250 bpm fall within the VF zone.

VF Zone

Sustained arrhythmias with rates sensed within the VF zone are detected as VF. However, not all arrhythmias within the VF zone are true VF. The rate limit for the VF zone is programmed to cover serious arrhythmias (at rates high enough to adversely affect the general status of the patient) that call for high-voltage therapies. In this zone, only high-voltage therapy is allowed.

VT Zone

Sustained arrhythmias within the VT zone are detected by the ICD as VT. Some devices allow for more than one VT zone, which allows for different therapies depending on the rate of the VT. The rate limit for VT is programmed to cover arrhythmic rates but not low enough to also cover elevated sinus rhythm. This may sometimes cause problems when the arrhythmia is slow and the sinus rate may reach rates above that of the arrhythmia. In these cases, the use of discriminators, which judge the rhythm by other criteria than rate alone, is called for. These algorithms may differentiate between rhythms and help to prevent therapy from being delivered on fast sinus rhythm. In the VT zone, the first therapies are commonly a few ATP sequences, with high-voltage therapy (cardioversion) following ATP if not successful.

FVT Zone

In ICDs from Medtronic, it is possible to program a zone for fast VT (FVT) that may be programmed via the VT or the VF zone. The zone chosen decides which counter will be used for FVT. The Medtronic VT counter demands consecutive intervals in the VT zone, while the VF counter is probabilistic and demands, for example, 12/16 intervals within the zone to detect arrhythmia. If activated, FVT via VF is by far the most common alternative.

Monitor Zone

In some ICDs, it is possible to program a zone for monitoring arrhythmia. In this zone, it is possible to monitor for slow, previously undetected arrhythmias without delivering therapy. An alternative in some models is to program a slow VT zone without therapies.

Detection Counters

An ICD needs to recognize and distinguish between many types of arrhythmias and to be able to discriminate, for example, atrial arrhythmia from ventricular arrhythmia. Different types of arrhythmias have diverse characteristics. As an example, VF is a rhythm that commonly exhibits a fast rate, relatively low amplitudes of intracardiac signals, and irregular intervals. These characteristics differ from the typical VT, which commonly has a lower rate than VF (longer VV intervals), higher intracardiac amplitudes, and more regular intervals. Supraventricular arrhythmias may result in a fast, regular ventricular rhythm (such as atrial flutter and other types of fast, regular atrial rhythms), or in a more irregular ventricular rhythm (such as atrial fibrillation). The rate and regularity of the resulting ventricular rhythm depends on AV nodal ability to conduct the fast signals from the atrium to the ventricle. AV blocks are commonly seen during fast atrial rates (2:1, Wenckebach, etc.).

As described earlier, ventricular rate needs to fall into one of the detection zones for arrhythmia detection to occur. Also, the arrhythmia needs to be sustained. Companies use various approaches to determine whether the arrhythmia is sustained. The most common way is to use some kind of counter that counts the number of beats within a detection zone. The actual number of beats is programmed separately for each detection zone. This approach is used by ICDs from Medtronic, St. Jude Medical, and Biotronik. Another way to determine whether the arrhythmia is sustained is to program a duration in seconds. The arrhythmia then needs to be ongoing for that amount of time to trigger therapy. However, with this approach a counter is also active to make sure that a large enough number of intervals falls within the zone during the programmed duration. This approach is used in ICDs from Boston Scientific.

The VT Counter

ICDs from Medtronic and Biotronik use a different type of counter for the VT and the VF zones. The counters are deliberately different due to the diverse characteristics of the arrhythmias expected in the respective zones. Arrhythmias found in the VT zone are generally regular with comparatively high intracardiac amplitudes. To detect this type of arrhythmia, the VT counter is designed to count *consecutive* intervals within the VT zone. A single long interval outside the detection zone will reset the counter to zero. Detection occurs when the programmed number of intervals is reached by the counter. ICDs from Boston Scientific and St. Jude Medical use the same type of counter for VT and VF. These do not reset on occasional long intervals.

The VT counter ensures that the arrhythmia is sustained and demands therapy. Short, non-sustained arrhythmias are allowed to self-terminate without intervention from the ICD. How long it is safe to wait before therapy is delivered differs between patients. Patients less tolerant of their arrhythmias should receive therapy earlier (after a smaller number of VT intervals), while patients more tolerant could wait somewhat longer to allow for possible self-termination. There is always a risk that the delivered therapy causes the arrhythmia to deteriorate, which in itself is a reason to not deliver therapy too soon.

The number of intervals needed to detect arrhythmia can be called, for example, number of intervals to detect, or NID.

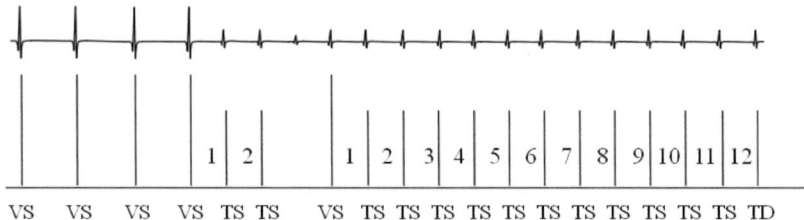

Figure 7.3 The VT-counter is a consecutive counter that is reset whenever an interval falls below the detection zone. In this example, undersensing of the third arrhythmia complex leads to reset of the counter to zero in a Medtronic ICD.

The VF Counter

Arrhythmias found within the VF zone may be fast, irregular, and with small or varying signal amplitudes (even though fast, regular VT is also often found in this zone). To better detect these types of arrhythmias, the VF counter in Medtronic and Biotronik ICDs is probabilistic. This means that occasional long intervals outside of the zone will not reset the counter. This is important since occasional long intervals are more commonly seen in these types of arrhythmias, and reset of the VF counter to zero would lead to unwanted prolongation of the time to detection. Programming of NID in the VF zone for Medtronic and Biotronik is done as for example 9/12, meaning that detection will occur when 9 out of 12 intervals are within the zone. In ICDs from St. Jude Medical, none of the counters are reset on occasional long intervals, and for Boston Scientific, both a counter and a duration need to be fulfilled.

Also in the VF zone, the decision needs to be made on how long it is safe to wait before therapy is delivered. Patients less tolerant of their arrhythmias should receive therapy earlier (after a smaller number of VF intervals), while patients more tolerant could wait somewhat longer to allow for possible self-termination. It is worth noting that also in the VF zone, the most common arrhythmia is fast VT! In VF it is important to start therapy as soon as possible to re-establish circulation. Chances for successful defibrillation decrease with time. However, longer detection time decreases the risk of inappropriate high-voltage therapy based on, for example, external noise or broken leads.

Also in the VF zone, the parameter is called number of intervals to detect, or NID.

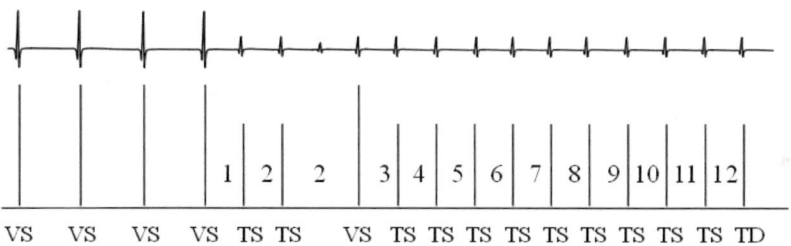

FIGURE 7.4 The VF counter is a probabilistic counter that demands, for example, 12/16 intervals to be within the VF zone to detect VF. In this example, undersensing of the third arrhythmia complex does not reset the counter, which instead stays at a value of 2.

Combined Count

It is not uncommon to see arrhythmias with intervals that alternate between the different detection zones, some in the VT and others in the VF zone. In order to speed up detection in those cases, the ICD will use some kind of combined count for detection. This could be, for example, a separate counter that keeps track of the total number of intervals in any detection zone, allowing for detection even though neither the VF nor the VT counters have fulfilled their NID.

Arrhythmia Confirmation

When an arrhythmia is detected in the VF zone, the ICD starts to charge the capacitors to deliver high-voltage therapy. The time to do so depends on the manufacturer, battery discharge, etc. Normal charge time is approximately 5 to 15 seconds, during which it is possible for the arrhythmia to self-terminate. To avoid delivery of high-voltage therapy after the arrhythmia has terminated, the ICD will check again to confirm that the arrhythmia is ongoing before therapy is delivered. This final check may be called confirmation or reconfirmation, depending on manufacturer. The manufacturers use different algorithms to confirm arrhythmias, but all are consistent in that to confirm an arrhythmia, short VV intervals need to be detected after or during capacitor charging.

Detection and Re-Detection

After detecting a ventricular arrhythmia (initial detection) and delivering therapy, the ICD continues to monitor heart-rate to ensure that the delivered therapy was successful. If this first therapy was not successful, the ICD will re-detect the arrhythmia. When this happens, it is important to deliver the next therapy as soon as possible to restore circulation. In a case when the first therapy was unsuccessful, the arrhythmia has already been ongoing for many seconds, and in order not to delay therapy more than necessary, NID (or duration) is programmed shorter for re-detection than for initial detection. It is also important to note that many of the discriminators against SVT are not active during re-detection.

Discriminators against SVT

Early ICDs were of a much simpler design than those of today, and based arrhythmia detection on ventricular rate alone. Today's ICDs incorporate much more sophisticated algorithms to decide whether a treatable ventricular arrhythmia is present. Ventricular rate naturally still plays an important role when investigating the rhythm, but rate alone cannot always discriminate between atrial and ventricular arrhythmia, where the latter normally should be treated while the first should not. Some of the characteristics that may differ in atrial and ventricular arrhythmia are:

- Start of the arrhythmia: In exercise-induced sinus tachycardia, the rate increase is gradual, while the rate increase in VT usually is very sudden. In other types of atrial arrhythmias (atrial flutter, atrial fibrillation, etc.), the start is abrupt, and these may not be differentiated from VT by looking at the way the rate increases.

- Regularity: In atrial fibrillation, the ventricular rhythm is often irregular, while in reentry type VT, the rhythm usually is very regular.
- Morphology: In rapidly conducted atrial tachycardia, the morphology of the ventricular complexes are usually the same as during sinus rhythm (narrow), while a VT often results in wider complexes.

It is of utmost importance that discriminators be available for the ICD to differentiate between atrial and ventricular arrhythmias to avoid inappropriate therapy. It is also extremely important that the ICD, if there is any doubt, always deliver therapy on a suspected life-threatening arrhythmia. We demand 100% sensitivity for detection of ventricular arrhythmia (i.e., all VT/VF are detected as arrhythmia) and this cannot be compromised. The discriminators used must give therapy one time too many rather than miss one real episode of arrhythmia. When discussing the algorithm's ability to correctly discriminate atrial arrhythmia and thereby inhibit therapy, we talk about specificity. There are no discrimination algorithms with 100% specificity. The Medtronic discriminator PRLogic, which has a very high specificity in this context, has a positive predicted value (proportion of positive test results that are true positives) of 78.1%.[8] By combining the discriminators, it is possible to increase specificity and minimize the risk of inappropriate therapies.

To increase specificity, some ICDs use a different EGM vector than for sensing for some of the discriminators. A more ECG-like signal may be achieved by using an extracardiac vector, such as SVC coil to can, and could be very useful for discriminators analyzing morphology. For a VT with wide QRSs on surface ECG, the morphology change on the bipolar vector may be marginal. However, when using an extracardiac vector, the

---

[8] Circulation 2001;103:381-6

changes are more pronounced since a larger part of ventricular polarization is covered and the signal is thus more ECG-like.

When discriminating against SVT, there is commonly a rate limitation up to which the discriminators are allowed to evaluate the rhythm. This can be a programmable rate (SVT limit) or can be linked to the rates of the highest detection zone (no discrimination in that zone).

It can also be of importance to understand how the discriminators interact and in which order they evaluate the rhythm. To inhibit therapy, do they all have to agree, or is it enough if one says SVT? Unfortunately this is very much manufacturer-specific and will therefore not be discussed in detail in this book.

Onset

For patients with slow VT and high sinus rate during exercise (within the VT zone), the ICD cannot discriminate VT from sinus rhythm just by analyzing the rate. To be able to give correct therapy for this patient population, one of the first discriminators, onset, was developed. This discriminator uses the fact that most VTs start abruptly, while an increase in sinus rate is more gradual. For example, a mean value from the last four intervals may be calculated and compared to the mean value for the previous four intervals. The result is compared to a programmable percentage (%) or a variance in ms, and can tell whether the rate acceleration was fast enough to indicate VT. A lower percentage means that a faster acceleration is needed to detect VT. Nominal value is around 80%.

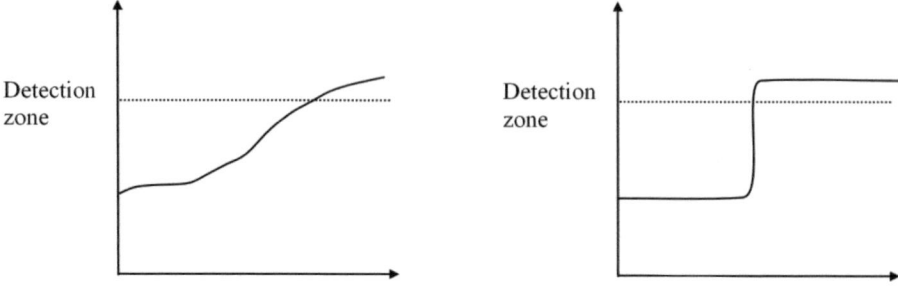

FIGURE 7.5 Discrimination using onset. Left: increasing sinus rhythm during exercise. The slow increase in heart-rate does not lead to arrhythmia detection, even though the rate falls within the detection zone. Right: abrupt increase in heart-rate that leads to detection of arrhythmia, and possibly therapy, when the rate falls within the detection zone.

If onset is used, it is important to remember that this kind of discriminator may decrease sensitivity for true ventricular arrhythmia, which is the reason why many experts advise against using it. Deaths have been reported in patients with exercise-induced VT where the comparatively small difference in rate may go undetected and the onset parameter therefore inhibits therapy. Activation of onset may also prevent more specific discriminators from evaluating the rhythm.

Re-detection: Onset discrimination can only be done when the rate accelerates into the detection zone. It is therefore not active during re-detection.

Stability

The most common cause of inappropriate therapy is atrial fibrillation. When the rhythm is rapidly conducted to the ventricle, the resulting ventricular rate is often within the detection zone. It is therefore not possible to discriminate between VT and AF by evaluating rate alone. Notable on surface ECG, however, is the difference in regularity between the two. In VT the rhythm is normally very stable with VV intervals varying by little more than a dozen milliseconds. However, in atrial fibrillation the rhythm is commonly irregular with large variance from interval to interval. This can be used by the ICD by looking at the stability between intervals. A value in milliseconds is programmed, and if the inter-interval difference is larger than that, the rhythm is detected as AF. There are some limitations to this type of algorithm, since the ventricular rhythm tends to be more regular at higher rates. It could still be useful in selected patients and is often used in single-chamber devices to minimize inappropriate therapy on AF.

Re-detection: Induction of AF is always a possibility when delivering high-voltage therapy. It is therefore important that the ICD be allowed to re-evaluate the rhythm after therapy. Hence, the stability discriminator is active during re-detection.

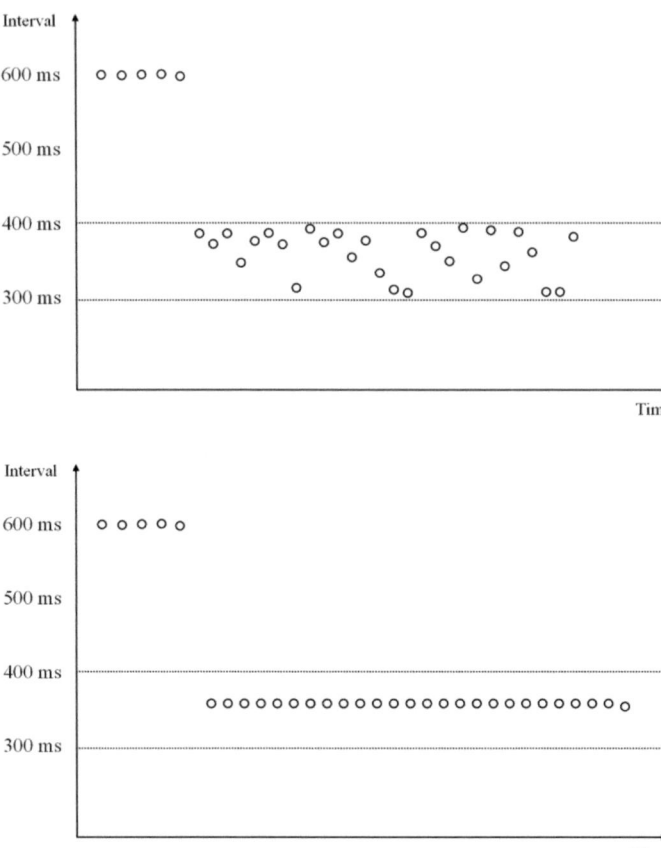

FIGURE 7.6 Top: atrial fibrillation with irregular ventricular response. This rhythm will not lead to therapy since the ICD, with stability, will interpret the irregular rhythm as AF. Bottom: VT resulting in a stable ventricular rhythm. With stability the ICD will interpret the regular rhythm as VT and will deliver therapy if the rhythm is sustained within the detection zone.

AV Analysis

When interpreting arrhythmia on surface ECG, it is often difficult, if not impossible, to evaluate the possible relation between atrium and ventricle. This is not the case, however, for an implanted dual-chamber ICD, which has access to information about both atrial and ventricular activity. It is therefore possible for the ICD to use the relation between atrium and ventricle when evaluating the rhythm. This can be done by using algorithms of varying complexity to decide whether the arrhythmia is initiated in atrium, and should not be treated, or in the ventricle, where therapy should be delivered. There are some similarities between the models but also substantial differences.

By comparing the rate in the atrium with that in the ventricle, the ICD can get a rough idea of what arrhythmia is occurring. If the ventricular rate is higher than that in the atrium, it is most likely a ventricular tachycardia, while a faster rate in the atrium indicates an atrial arrhythmia that is being rapidly conducted to the ventricles. If the rates are similar, it is more difficult and could be either an atrial tachycardia or a 1:1 retrograde conducting VT.

The companies St. Jude Medical (Rate Branch), Biotronik (SMART Detection), and Boston Scientific all have algorithms that calculate a mean or median rate for the atrium as well as for the ventricle and compare the two. Depending on the result, another discriminator may or may not be indicated (stability, onset, and in some cases morphology). As an example, an atrial rate that is faster than the ventricular rate may lead to a second opinion from the stability discriminator, or a morphologic comparison may be made, before therapy can be delivered.

In the Medtronic ICDs, a somewhat more sophisticated analysis is used, called PRLogic (pattern recognition). This discriminator monitors every heart cycle looking for patterns that may help characterize the arrhythmia. The number of atrial events between ventricular events is noted, as well as their relation to the ventricular signals. The algorithm analyzes rates, stability, and AV association, as well as signs of FFRW oversensing. A somewhat similar but slightly less advanced algorithm is the St. Jude Medical AV Association.

Morphology

The majority of modern ICDs have the ability to analyze the morphology of the ventricular complex and compare it to a reference complex collected during sinus rhythm. These algorithms are based on the fact that true VT normally has a wider QRS than that of sinus rhythm, while conducted atrial arrhythmias usually lack those changes (except for rate-dependent bundle branch block). This discriminator is especially useful in single-chamber ICDs, where monitoring of the atrial rhythm is not possible.

Morphological analysis may be performed either on the near-field EGM (bipolar or integrated) or on a far-field EGM (for example, SVC coil to can). The largest change in morphology can be seen in the more ECG-like far-field signal, but the companies use different technologies and algorithms. It is important to make sure that the vector used for morphology discrimination is correctly programmed.

For morphology discrimination to work, the ICD needs to store a reference complex during sinus rhythm for comparison with the morphology during the arrhythmia. This reference complex is collected and stored when the algorithm is activated during ICD follow-up, after which most devices may be updated automatically, either at pre-set intervals or continuously if the morphology changes and no longer matches the reference. Different companies have different solutions for this.

Collection of the reference complex needs to be done on intrinsic QRS, not during pacemaker stimulation. The algorithm may therefore be of less use for pacemaker-dependent patients or for patients treated with a CRT-D device.

For patients with rate-dependent bundle branch block (BBB), the automatic update of the reference complex cannot be used, since the morphology is expected to change for elevated sinus rhythm as well and thus would be interpreted as VT. To work around this, it is possible to do a manual collection of the reference complex during exercise and then switch off the automatic updates. When the rate reaches the detection zone, the ICD will compare the morphology to the collected one (with BBB), and a deviant morphology during VT will result in therapy.

Morphological discriminators include, for example, Wavelet (Medtronic), Morphology Discrimination (St. Jude Medical), and Rhythm Match (Boston Scientific).

Re-detection: Morphology discrimination can only be used during primary detection since the morphology often changes immediately after high-voltage therapy.

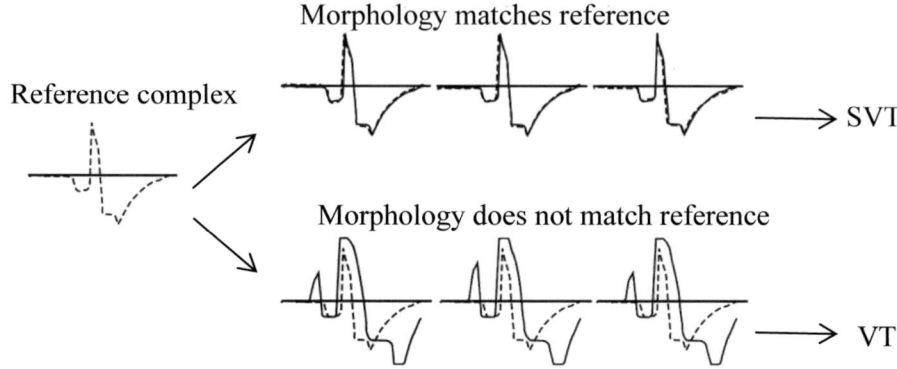

FIGURE 7.7 SVT discrimination with morphology (Medtronic Wavelet). The complexes found in the detection zone are compared to the reference complex collected during sinus rhythm. If they are morphologically equivalent, the ICD will interpret the rhythm as SVT and inhibit therapy.

Other Discriminators

In addition to discrimination between SVT and VT, it is desirable that the ICD also be able to discriminate between VT and various types of oversensing. The most commonly seen types of oversensing are T wave oversensing and oversensing of signals created by a fractured sensing lead (lead noise).

T Wave Discrimination

The input amplifier of the ICD incorporates a bandpass filter that only lets signals of a certain frequency content to pass though. Since the frequency content of the T wave is usually lower than that of the R wave, T waves are filtered out and do not reach the sensing amplifier, while R waves pass though unchanged. Unfortunately, this is not true for all situations, and some patients may temporarily, or more permanently, exhibit pathological T waves with a frequency content close to that of the R wave. This may cause serious problems with double sensing that at higher sinus rates may lead to inappropriate detection and therapy. In addition to the previously described strategies to deal with T wave oversensing (sensitivity, decay delay, sensing polarity, new pace/sense lead), new algorithms designed primarily to differentiate R waves from T waves have recently reached the market (for example, Medtronic T wave discrimination). This can be done safely without changing the sensitivity by analyzing amplitude and interval relationship after additional frequency analysis to separate R waves from T waves. If the rhythm fulfills all criteria for T wave oversensing, detection is inhibited and inappropriate therapy can be avoided.

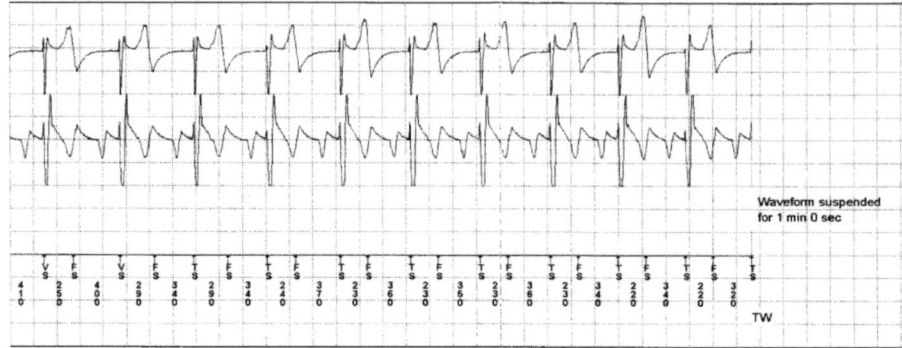

FIGURE 7.8 T wave oversensing in a Medtronic Protecta VR device. Upper curve shows bipolar EGM (RV tip to RV ring). Lower curve shows an extracardiac vector between RV coil and SVC coil (leadless ECG). Note the large T waves that are sensed by the device and marked with FS. When the detection counter reaches its programmed value, the TWOS algorithm will analyze the signals and, in this case, interpret the rhythm as sinus rhythm with T wave oversensing. Detection is held back, and the rhythm is marked with TW in the marker channel.

Lead Noise Discrimination

Electrical signals generated by a faulty or incorrectly connected lead are often seen in showers and may be detected at a very high rate well into the VF detection zone. These showers of noise are often the first sign of a failing lead and could very quickly lead to inappropriate and repeated high-voltage therapies. When this happens, the patient needs to get to the hospital as soon as possible for deactivation of the system and replacement of the lead. To prevent this type of noise from causing inappropriate therapy, there are specific algorithms in some ICDs that are designed to monitor for signs of lead failure by comparing the signals seen on the near-field EGM (bipolar or integrated) with the ones on the far-field EGM (RV coil to can). These signals should match as long as the sensed signals originate in the ventricle, but differ when the signals are artifacts from a fractured lead. By triggering an alarm when lead noise is detected, the patient may escape inappropriate therapy and seek medical care in time to have the problem fixed before it gets serious.

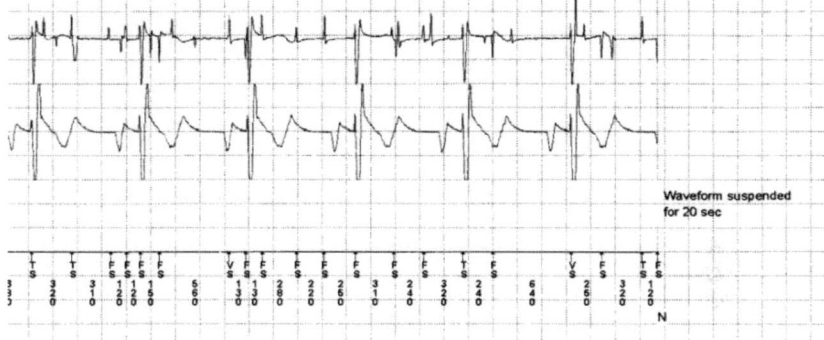

Waveform suspended
for 20 sec

FIGURE 7.9 Medtronic Protecta VR. Noise from a faulty lead can be seen as showers of signals on the bipolar (upper) tracing. Since these signals are not found in the lower RV coil to SVC coil tracing, the ICD interprets this (correctly) as being lead noise, withholds detection, and marks the rhythm with an N (noise) in the marker channel.

Tachy Therapies

When programming an ICD, some of the most fundamental parameters are those deciding the type of therapy to be delivered for different types of arrhythmia. There are differences between ATP therapies (anti-tachy pacing, low-voltage therapy) and defibrillation/cardioversion (high-voltage therapy). While ATP therapy is the first choice for most regular, reentry tachycardia (pain-free, energy-saving, and often effective), high-voltage therapy is used for faster VT and ventricular fibrillation. High-voltage therapy may be very painful when delivered to a conscious patient, but for some arrhythmias, it cannot be avoided. It is also important to remember that although the therapy is delivered to normalize heart rhythm, it may in some cases cause it to deteriorate. Modern ICDs are capable of delivering several therapies within each detection zone. If more than one therapy is needed, the ICD usually starts with the less aggressive ones and becomes more aggressive for each new therapy delivered (except for in the VF zone, where usually only shocks with maximum energy are delivered).

ATP Therapies

In reentry arrhythmia, delivery of ATP therapy is often found to be successful in terminating the arrhythmia. ATP therapy is delivered as a pulse train of low-voltage pacemaker pulses in the heart chamber where the reentry circuitry is localized. This is a totally pain-free treatment, unlike high-voltage therapy, and in addition requires less energy. Also, arrhythmias of a rather high rate may be safely terminated with ATP, and it is not uncommon in modern devices to be able to program ATP therapies to be delivered in the VF zone also. This may be done by allowing the ICD to deliver ATP simultaneously with capacitor charging to deliver high-voltage therapy (for example, Medtronic ATP during charging). If ATP is successful, charging and/or delivery of high-voltage therapy will be aborted.

ATP is only likely to be successful in certain types of arrhythmias such as reentry tachycardia. As described earlier, the substrate for reentry tachycardia is dual, parallel pathways around a central conduction block. The pathways must be connected at both ends and exhibit different characteristics. One pathway needs to have fast conduction time and prolonged refractory periods, while the other needs to reverse that by having a slow conduction time with short refractory. During the arrhythmia, the depolarization wave will follow the reentry circuit and create feedback which will facilitate and maintain the high, non-physiologic rate. During this feedback, there is always a small part of the reentry that is not refractory and, as such, may be depolarized again. This short window is called the gap of excitability. If a pacemaker-induced depolarization wave can activate this non-refractory window in the reentry circuit, the arrhythmia may be terminated. However, the window is very short, and to capture the substrate, the ICD stimulates at a rate slightly higher than that of the arrhythmia. By gradually taking over more and more of the ventricular activation, the ATP sequence will eventually also capture the substrate and terminate the arrhythmia. The intervals between the pulses in the ATP sequence are programmed as a percentage of the arrhythmia interval. With an arrhythmia rate of 210 bpm, the arrhythmia interval equals 286 ms. For ATP delivered at 88% of the arrhythmia interval, therapy will be delivered at 250 ms.

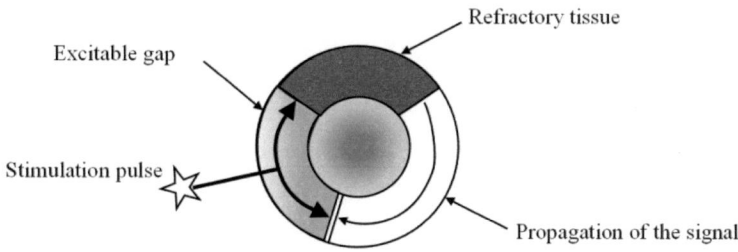

FIGURE 8.1 In order to terminate a tachycardia using ATP, one or more of the delivered stimulation pulses need to capture the gap of excitability. When this happens, the resulting depolarization will split at the site of the conduction block, and if successful, one branch will meet refractory tissue and the other will cause refractory that will collide with depolarization of the reentry circuit and terminate the arrhythmia.

When stimulating in close proximity to the absolute physiological refractory of the tissue, higher energy levels are commonly needed to achieve capture. In addition, during arrhythmia, heart perfusion may be compromised, which may also lead to an increased threshold. Stimulation output is therefore commonly programmed to higher values for the ATP pulses than for bradycardia pacing.

Two different types of ATP protocols are available: burst and ramp. In a burst, every pulse is delivered at the same interval as the one before, while in a ramp, the pulses are delivered at decreasing intervals between pulses. Ramp protocols are often seen as slightly more aggressive. When more than one therapy is programmed (which is almost always), it is advised to use both ramp and burst protocols to increase the chance of successful termination of the arrhythmia. However, it is important to remember that ATP therapy may cause the arrhythmia to deteriorate. For poorly tolerated arrhythmias in the VT zone, it is always advised to program some of the (final) therapies for high-voltage cardioversion.

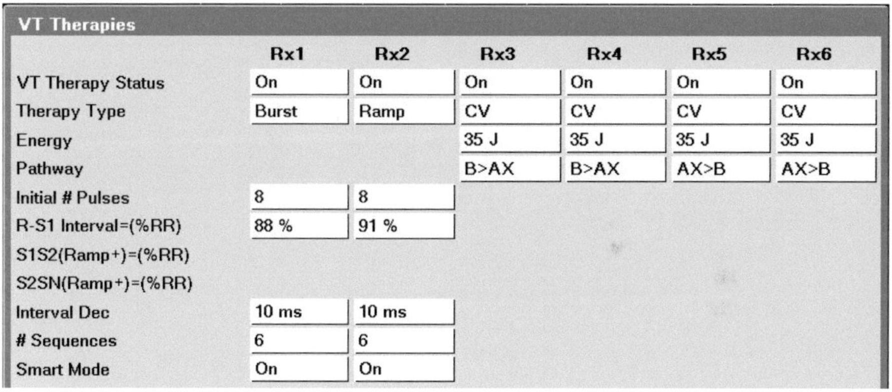

VT Therapies						
	Rx1	Rx2	Rx3	Rx4	Rx5	Rx6
VT Therapy Status	On	On	On	On	On	On
Therapy Type	Burst	Ramp	CV	CV	CV	CV
Energy			35 J	35 J	35 J	35 J
Pathway			B>AX	B>AX	AX>B	AX>B
Initial # Pulses	8	8				
R-S1 Interval=(%RR)	88 %	91 %				
S1S2(Ramp+)=(%RR)						
S2SN(Ramp+)=(%RR)						
Interval Dec	10 ms	10 ms				
# Sequences	6	6				
Smart Mode	On	On				

FIGURE 8.2 Programmer screen from a Medtronic Protecta ICD with therapies programmed for the VT zone.

Burst Therapy

A burst sequence is a train of pulses delivered at the same inter-pulse interval. The number of pulses delivered in the burst is programmable, as well as the relation between the arrhythmia intervals and the intervals of the burst (as a percentage of the arrhythmia interval). When programming burst therapy, the number of sequences also has to be defined, as well as the interval decrement if more than one sequence needs to be delivered. The latter is important since delivery of an identical burst after the first one will most likely lead to the same result. Shortening the interval with every new burst increases the chance of finding the most successful interval for the particular arrhythmia.

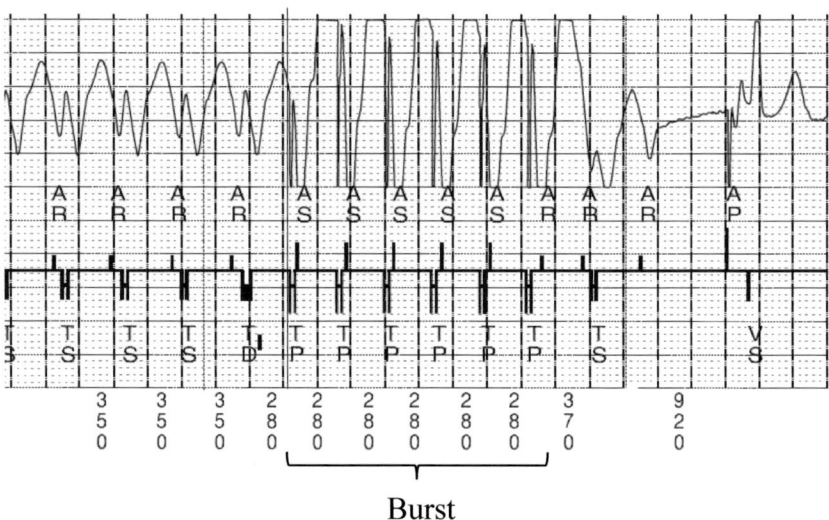

Burst

FIGURE 8.3 VT with a VV interval of 350 ms. Burst therapy is delivered at 81% of the arrhythmia interval with 6 pulses, which terminates the arrhythmia.

Ramp Therapy

Ramp therapy differs from burst therapy in that every interval in the ramp is shorter than the preceding one. The number of pulses is programmable, as are the first interval (as a percentage of the arrhythmia interval), the interval decrement per pulse, and the number of ramp sequences in the therapy. If therapy was not successful, a change needs to be made for the next sequence. This is often done by adding an extra pulse to the original pulse-train or by shortening the intervals.

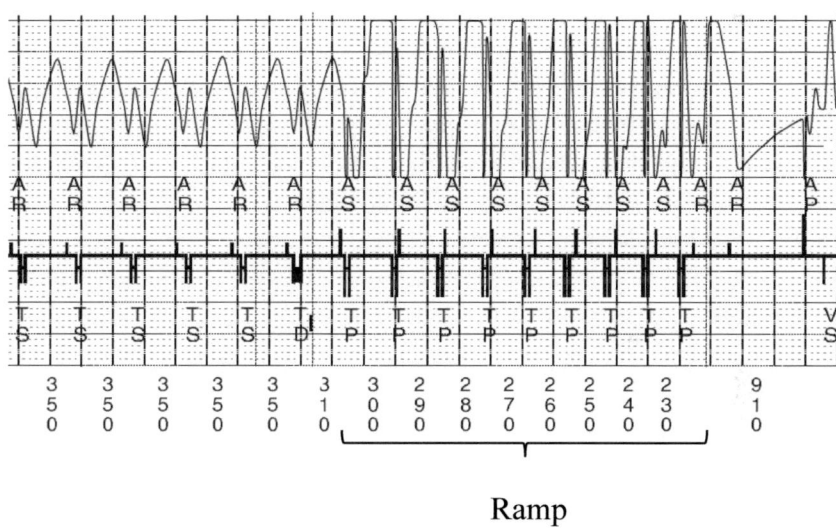

Ramp

FIGURE 8.4 VT with a VV interval of 350 ms. Ramp therapy is delivered at 88% of the arrhythmia VV interval at 9 pulses and an interval decrement of 10 ms between pulses.

Defibrillation

For arrhythmias where ATP therapy is not enough—for example, ventricular fibrillation—the use of high-voltage therapy (defibrillation) is necessary. High-voltage therapy may be programmed for all detection zones and is the only therapy available in the highest rate zone (VF zone), except for models with ATP during charging. If a VT zone is programmed, high-voltage therapy is often used for the last two or three therapies should ATP not be successful. Defibrillation energy is almost exclusively programmed to the highest energy (in Joules, J). In a few models on the market, the highest energy is not available until the second shock. The time from the start of the arrhythmia to delivery of the high-voltage therapy depends on the programmed NID, or detection time, and the charge time of the high-voltage capacitors. After detection and charging of the capacitors, the ICD re-confirms that the arrhythmia is ongoing and, if so, delivers defibrillation synchronized to a sensed ventricular event. This is important since a majority of the arrhythmias treated with high-voltage therapy, even in the VF zone, are actually VT. Synchronization of the energy to a ventricular complex lessens the risk for arrhythmia acceleration or deterioration into VF.

Other programmable defibrillation parameters may be the tilt of the pulse and the pulse configuration. The configuration may be, for example, RV coil to can. In some systems it is also possible to program the start polarity of the pulse, i.e., whether the coil or the can starts as the anode.

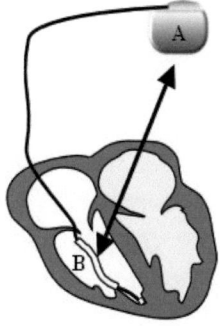 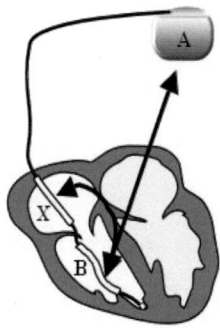

FIGURE 8.5 Left: energy is delivered between RV coil (B) and Active can (A) with a single-coil lead. Right: energy is delivered between RV coil (B) and Active can/SVC (AX) with a dual-coil lead.

Inappropriate Therapies

Although modern ICDs are equipped with sophisticated algorithms to discriminate ventricular arrhythmias from atrial arrhythmias or external noise, the problem of patients receiving high-voltage therapy without life-threatening arrhythmia still exists. However, the proportion of patients suffering from inappropriate therapies is decreasing with the development of new and more effective discrimination algorithms. We differentiate between unnecessary and inappropriate therapies.

When a patient receives high-voltage therapy for a ventricular arrhythmia within the detection zone that would have terminated spontaneously had a higher NID (longer detection time) been programmed, or where ATP therapy would have been successful, the term *unnecessary* therapy is used. It is, of course, often impossible to know whether high-voltage therapy

103

could have been avoided with a different programming strategy, but a modern ICD should allow for at least one sequence of ATP, even at higher rates, and, if the clinical status of the patient allows for it, a somewhat prolonged detection time to allow for self-termination whenever possible.

Inappropriate therapy is high-voltage therapy delivered when no ventricular arrhythmia is present. The most common cause for inappropriate therapy is atrial arrhythmias (with a fast ventricular response) and various types of oversensing (T wave oversensing, lead noise, or external electrical noise).

Delivery of high-voltage therapy is totally out of the patient's control and can also be very painful. In false detection it is not uncommon for the patient to receive repeated therapies since the cause for detection is not eliminated by the therapy. For some patients this may lead to great fear of this happening again, resulting in a decreased quality of life. It is important to identify these patients at an early stage and help them feel safe with their ICD. Cognitive behavioral therapy (CBT) can make a big difference, and it is advantageous to have an established cooperation between the cardiologist and a CBT therapist experienced in this field. Correctly delivered therapy can also cause very strong anxiety and angst since it reminds patients of their mortality. These patients may benefit from CBT as well.

SVT

Supraventricular tachycardia—for example, atrial fibrillation—is the most common cause of inappropriate delivery of high-voltage therapy. The ICD is equipped with various discrimination algorithms to differentiate between SVT and VT, as described earlier. However, none of these have a specificity of 100%. The most common causes for inappropriate therapy are described below.

SVT limit too low: This is a programmable rate limit that determines whether or not discrimination algorithms are allowed to evaluate the rhythm. For arrhythmias with rates above SVT limit, only the rate criteria is used for detection, which may lead to SVTs with a fast ventricular response being detected as VT/VF.

Solution: Increase SVT limit to allow the discriminators to evaluate the rhythm.

Fast and regular AV conduction: In a single-chamber ICD, information about the atrial rate is not available. With the stability discriminator activated, the ventricular rate needs to be irregular to inhibit detection. Unfortunately, this is not always the case, and for SVTs resulting in a fast and regular ventricular rate, stability is not effective.

Solution: If available, activate a morphology discriminator that will inhibit detection if no change in QRS morphology from the registered sinus rhythm is detected.

Atrial flutter with 1:1 conduction: This rhythm is difficult even for dual-chamber discriminators. Differentiating VT with 1:1 retrograde conduction from SVT with 1:1 antegrade conduction can be almost impossible, even during manual ECG interpretation. Onset is of no use since atrial flutter often has an abrupt start. Stability is not successful due to the regular ventricular rate, and even PRLogic has a hard time since the pattern can be identical for the two scenarios.

Solution: If available, activate a morphology discriminator that will inhibit detection if no change in QRS morphology from the registered sinus rhythm is detected.

Rate-dependent bundle branch block: For patients developing bundle branch block at increased heart rates, morphological discriminators may not be effective since QRS morphology changes not only during VT but also during fast atrial rhythm. This may lead to arrhythmia detection and therapy if the ventricular rate is fast enough to fall within a detection zone.

Solution: If morphology discrimination is desired, some systems may be programmed to compare QRS morphology with one that has been collected during exercise and therefore exhibits the broader morphology. The reference complex is collected while the patient does an exercise test on bicycle or treadmill and is then stored as a fixed value—i.e., no automaticity is switched on to update the reference over time. Since the discriminator is only active in a detection zone, sinus rhythm at lower rates will not be affected. It is important to make sure that the change in morphology takes place at a lower rate than the lower rate-limit for VT in order not to cause detection on the narrower complexes when the rate enters the detection zone.

Atrial under- or oversensing: Some discriminators are built on algorithms that compare ventricular and atrial rhythm. If the atrial rate is faster than the ventricular rate, atrial arrhythmia or dual (atrial and ventricular) arrhythmia is detected. If atrial sensing is not correct, the ICD may be misled, leading to inappropriate therapy. It is therefore important that the ICD correctly senses both the atrium and the ventricle.

Solution: The same as for other sensing problems: Reprogramming of sensitivity or repositioning/replacement of the atrial lead.

T Wave Oversensing (TWOS)

An ICD, similar to a pacemaker, has filters on the input amplifier to differentiate between R waves and T waves. The T wave commonly has a lower frequency content than the R wave, which leads to a decrease in amplitude when passing through the filter, while the QRS complex passes through unaffected. However, some patients have T waves with a frequency content very close to that of the R wave. In these cases, the T wave signal will be of high amplitude even after the filter, sometimes high enough to cross the sensitivity level. It is not uncommon that the T wave changes in morphology due to ischemia, caused by an increased heart rate during exercise. This may be difficult to predict, and TWOS is therefore often not discovered until after the first inappropriate therapy.

Solution: A couple of different strategies may be tried. If the ICD has a specific algorithm against TWOS, this should naturally be switched on. Careful evaluation of the EGM signals may indicate whether the problem can be solved by reprogramming sensitivity (lower sensitivity = higher value in mV). For this approach to be successful, the filtered R wave needs to be significantly larger than that of the T wave. It is also important to take into account that a lower sensitivity may lead to problems detecting real VF. Another possible solution is to reprogram the sensing polarity. This cannot be done with all ICDs, but when available, a change from bipolar to integrated sensing may prove effective. In some ICDs the decay curve that the sensing follows after a ventricular event may be changed, a parameter called decay delay. A prolongation of the decay delay may decrease the risk for TWOS but may at the same time possibly increase the risk for undersensing of arrhythmia. The last, and invasive, solution is to reposition the RV lead or to add an extra sense/pace lead beside the ICD lead. Ideally, a more optimal position with less ischemia and less prominent T waves can be found. Whichever solution is used, it is important to let the patient perform an exercise test afterward with ICD detection or therapy switched off so the EGM and markers can be closely monitored for signs of TWOS. If TWOS is still observed, the action taken was not sufficient, and additional changes are needed to avoid delivery of more inappropriate therapies.

P Wave Oversensing

When programmed for integrated sensing polarity, the ICD measures the difference in potential between RV tip and RV coil. For this to work safely, it is important that the RV coil not protrude into the atrium. If the coil is too long or not placed apically enough, P waves may be sensed on the ventricular channel, possibly leading to detection and inappropriate therapy.

Solution: If possible, the sensing polarity should be reprogrammed to be bipolar. Unfortunately, it is often impossible to solve the problem by reprogramming sensitivity since the timing of the P wave coincides with the part of the heart cycle when the ICD has the highest sensitivity (lowest value). Repositioning of the lead may be the only solution.

Non-Physiologic Oversensing

The task of an ICD is primarily to sense small electrical signals that occur with a high rate between the electrodes in the heart. To discriminate between heart signals and other types of electrical signals, the ICD is equipped with an electronic filter which favors signals with the "right" frequency content. There is, unfortunately, no guarantee that other electrical signals (interference) are not occasionally sensed, leading to inappropriate therapy. There are two types of interference that are responsible for the majority of these problems:

- Defect, or incorrectly connected, pace/sense lead
- External noise

Connector/lead problems are the more common of the two.

Defect pace/sense lead: An ICD lead is constructed from a number of conductors (two conductors for bipolar pace/sense, one conductor for the RV coil, and possibly also one additional for the SVC coil). These are coil-shaped and run in parallel inside the insulation. Each coil is constructed from a number of thinner conductors. If the lead is subject to excessive mechanical force, these thin conductors may start to fracture. When this happens to any of the two conductors used for sensing, movement of the lead may cause the surfaces of fracture to make intermittent contact, which in turn leads to small electrical signals. If these signals exceed the sensitivity level, inappropriate detection and therapy might be the result.

Solution: Once the problem occurs, there is only one solution, namely to switch off the ICD (or to switch off detection) and to monitor the patient until the lead is replaced. When it comes to preventive programming to avoid inappropriate therapy should the lead fail, there are a handful of solutions that together will give the patient relatively good, but not 100%, protection. The intention of these algorithms is to warn the patient/physician when something is wrong and, by doing so, increase the chance that the problem is corrected before inappropriate therapy is delivered. Various types of alerts, preferably combined with remote monitoring, will give an early warning. It is important that the system react not only to changes in impedance, since partial fraction may not lead to significant impedance changes, but also to signs of oversensing. These may manifest as short showers of noise registered by the ICD as non-sustained

VT but also, as is the case with ICDs from Medtronic, as an increased number of SIC (sensing integrity counter) events. This counter monitors sensed events with very short, non-physiologic, V-to-V intervals (< 130 ms). In a Medtronic ICD, these three parameters (impedance, non-sustained VT, and SIC) are monitored by a safety algorithm called LIA (lead integrity alert) that will give an alert at the first signs of a lead failure. This algorithm has been proven to decrease the number of patients receiving inappropriate high-voltage therapy caused by lead failure. As a result, 75% of patients will have at least three days to get to a hospital and have their system deactivated before inappropriate therapy starts to be delivered.[9]

Some of the newer systems have algorithms specifically designed to deal with noise from failing leads to avoid inappropriate therapy. For example, Medtronic Protecta was the first ICD to compare far-field EGM to near-field (bipolar or integrated). Signals detected only on the near-field EGM do not originate from the heart but rather represent noise from a fractured lead. By ignoring signals that cannot be detected on the far-field EGM as well, the device can differentiate between heart signals and noise.

Incorrect connection of the lead: At the time of implant, it is extremely important that the connection between the lead and the ICD be made correctly. Each lead connector pin should be inserted all the way to the end of the ICD connector block, and the set-screws should be tightened in such a way that the lead makes good contact with the ICD.

If any of the steps above should fail, the system will not function correctly with oversensing, undersensing, or inappropriate therapy as the result.

Solution: Diagnosing the problem may be done through X-ray of the ICD pocket, whereby it might be possible to see whether the connector pin is

[9] Circulation 2008;118:2122-9

fully inserted into the connector block. Lead impedance may vary a great deal, or the patient may already have received inappropriate therapy. Stored episodes of non-sustained VT and high SIC counts (Medtronic) may be present. The problem cannot be solved without surgery, where the connector should be carefully inspected and the lead pulled *before* the set-screw is touched.

External noise: Strong electromagnetic fields in the patient's environment may, in rare cases, generate enough noise in the lead to be sensed by ICD circuitry. Also, current leakage from, for example, a faulty floor-heating system, especially in the presence of water as an electric conductor, may cause inappropriate therapy. One example is a patient who received high-voltage therapy in a therapeutic bath (somewhat ironic maybe!), and another patient in whom the ICD detected a large amount of noise while showering in a building where the grounding system was faulty.

Solution: Unfortunately, the only solution is to recommend that the patient avoid the source of noise. If the noise was caused by malfunction in an electric system or appliance, this needs to be corrected immediately.

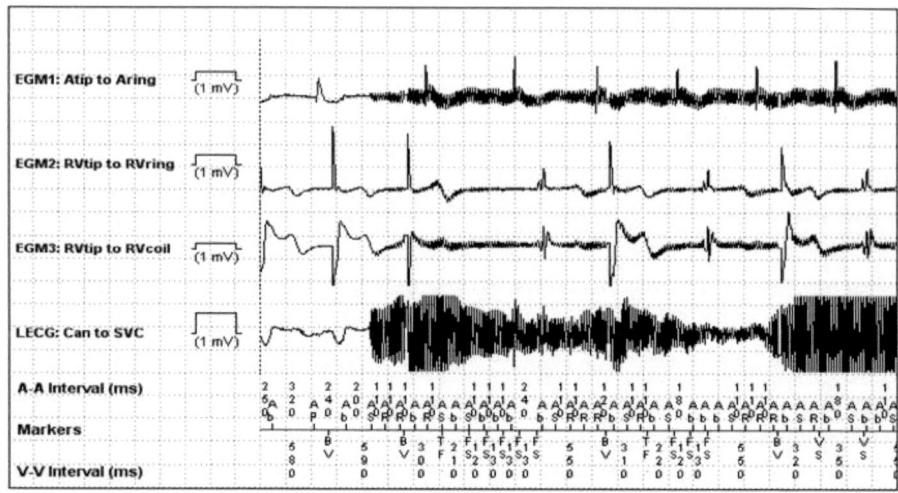

FIGURE 8.6 Stored episode from a Medtronic Maximo II CRT-D device. The patient is in his home showering. The noise is found to originate from faulty grounding in the bathroom. Fortunately, this did not lead to therapy since the signals are sensed intermittently in combination with initial NID programmed to 30/40.

The Implantation

The surgical implant procedure for an ICD doesn't differ much from that of a pacemaker. However, testing the system at the end of the implantation has until now been different and also demanded anesthesia. To make sure that the leads are in optimal positions to defibrillate the patient if needed, VF has been induced and the ICD has been allowed to detect and treat the arrhythmia. This test method is being used less and less in Europe, and is expected to decrease also in the U.S. which will facilitate the procedure. For patients with a severely reduced cardiac function, the induction of VF is risky and should in most cases be avoided. When this book was written, the SIMPLE trial (Shockless IMPLant Evaluation) was recently presented, in which 2500 patients were randomized to either DFT testing or no DFT testing at implantation. In this noninferiority trial the primary endpoint edged lower for patients randomized to no DFT testing. The results were very robust and are likely to change our practice to no DFT testing in the future.

It is however important to note that if we do not deliver a high-voltage pulse during the testing of the device, we may miss important information about lead integrity.

Before the start of the implantation, it is important that external defibrillation patches be attached to the patient. These are placed in such a way that the incision area is kept free. Anterior-posterior placement is preferred to avoid tissue damage around the lead tip should external defibrillation be necessary once the ICD lead is in place, but patches cannot be allowed to affect visibility of the heart on X-ray. The patches are connected to the external defibrillator, which should be switched on during the whole procedure.

Battery, Time, and Test Charge

Before the ICD is implanted, there are a few things that need to be tested. Making a habit of performing them in the same order every time will speed up the process and minimize the risk of missing any of the tasks. Remember never to switch on detection before the leads are connected and the ICD is placed in the pocket under the skin. It is very likely that the noise created by manipulating the device and lead connector will otherwise lead to high-voltage therapy!

The following steps may be followed when performing a technical check of the ICD before it is implanted:

1. Interrogate the ICD and check battery voltage. Battery voltage decreases if the ICD is cold but should read BOS voltage at room temperature. Never implant an ICD with lower battery voltage than that recommended by the manufacturer.
2. Check the clock and adjust for correct time and date if necessary.
3. For ICDs with capacitors needing reformation, a test charge should be performed. Check that the charge time is within normal values for the model/manufacturer. Let the voltage slowly dissolve (don't make an energy dump) in order to fully reform the capacitors.

Measurements

Once the leads are in place, measurements are taken for sensing, pacing thresholds, and impedances. This is done with an analyzer in the same way as during a pacemaker implantation. However, it is of very high importance that the amplitude of the R wave be as high as possible to ensure proper sensing during ventricular fibrillation and to avoid TWOS. An acute R wave of > 5 mV is desirable. This may seem like a high value since the sensitivity is commonly programmed to 0.3 mV, but it is not uncommon for the R wave to decrease somewhat after the implant. High amplitude is an indication of viable tissue around the lead tip, which may be predictive of good sensing also during VF.

Current of Injury

When a lead is positioned in the heart, it will damage some of the heart cells in contact with the lead tip, which will lead to a leakage of ions over the cell membranes. This is called current of injury and may be observed on the intracardiac registration as a characteristic distortion of signal morphology. This distortion is temporary but will affect the reading of the R wave such that the amplitude measurement may give a value that is too high. To ensure that the measured R wave amplitude is correct, the EGM signal should be evaluated closely. If current of injury is suspected of affecting the measured signal, the measurements should be taken again after a couple of minutes.

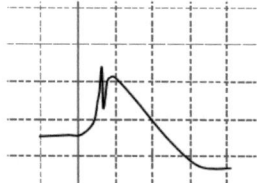 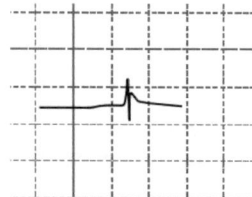

FIGURE 9.1 Current of injury at implantation. Left: measurement taken early after lead fixation showing a substantial current of injury. Right: same signal 10 minutes later when current of injury is almost completely gone.

Measurements with the ICD

Once acceptable values have been achieved for sensing, thresholds, and impedances using the analyzer, the leads are connected to the ICD. To make sure that the connections have been made correctly, the measurements are repeated with the ICD to confirm the values from the analyzer. Note that the sensing amplitude of the R wave may differ somewhat between measurements taken with the analyzer and those taken with the device. This is due to the fact that the device and the analyzer may use different filters and/or divergent measuring methods. Check carefully that there are no double-counting sense markers that may interfere with ICD detection of arrhythmia, and that thresholds and impedances are within expectations. Unfortunately, impedances within the normal range for the *high-voltage* leads do not guarantee correct connection. Some problems don't reveal themselves until delivery of high-voltage therapy.

Induction

Induction and conversion of VF is still performed as a routine test during ICD implantation in most centers in the U.S. In many countries in Europe, this test is no longer done routinely unless a high DFT can be expected, such as for right-sided implants, or if the patient is on Cordarone (Amiodarone). Recently presented results from the SIMPLE trial (Shockless IMPLant Evaluation) is likely to change this practice also in the U.S. In the SIMPLE trial 2500 patients were randomized to either DFT testing or no DFT testing at implantation. The primary endpoint for the study (the composite of failed shock for VT or VF or arrhythmic death) edged lower for patients in the non-DFT tested group.

As described earlier, not all high-voltage issues can be detected using low-voltage measurements. To discover possible lead damage that may have occurred since the previous implant, it is also desirable to deliver a high-voltage shock during a replacement procedure to make sure that the impedance is measured correctly. This is especially true for systems that have never delivered high-voltage therapy and therefore have not measured high-voltage impedance. Naturally, this can only be done during anesthesia. By inducing ventricular fibrillation and letting the ICD convert the arrhythmia, we get the following information:

- Is the device sensing correctly during ventricular fibrillation?
- Are the lead-device high-voltage connections correct?
- Is the high-voltage lead integrity OK?
- Is the ICD likely to convert ventricular fibrillation with the chosen lead configuration?

As described in an earlier chapter, the chance of converting ventricular fibrillation is probabilistic—i.e., if repeated inductions are performed and the same therapy is delivered every time, some therapies will be successful at terminating VF and others will not. Therefore, successful defibrillation in the operating theater is no guarantee for success later on. Threshold measurements like the ones done for pacemakers are not possible. Instead, the method of choice is commonly to use a LED (lowest energy delivered) test where the tested energy, if successful, indicates a certain safety margin when the ICD is programmed to its maximum energy. A DFT (defibrillation threshold) test out the real energy needed to defibrillate the heart. During a DFT test, repeated inductions are performed (usually at least three) where a different energy is delivered after each induction in order to discover the DFT. As mentioned earlier, this is not a completely reliable method since DFT is probabilistic.

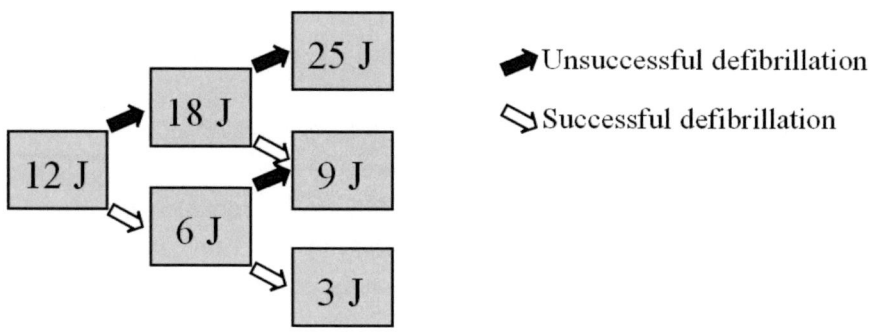

FIGURE 9.2 Binary VF induction search protocol to estimate DFT.

Before induction, the ICD is programmed in such a way that sensing and therapy can be evaluated. Sensitivity is commonly programmed to a higher value (lower sensitivity) than the permanent value used after the test. This helps determine the safety margin for sensing once the permanent value is programmed. Commonly, a value of four times the permanent value is used, which means a test value of 1.2 mV if the ICD is later to be programmed to a permanent value of 0.3 mV. If the device senses correctly during ventricular fibrillation, a safety margin of at least four times is achieved at a permanent sensitivity of 0.3 mV.

Before the induction, detection must be switched on and the VF zone needs to be defined. The rate limit should be programmed to around 300 ms to ensure proper detection and delivery of therapy for VF. It is desirable not to program a detection zone low enough to also cover possible slow VT. Should monomorphic VT be induced, there is no significant value in converting this arrhythmia with defibrillation therapy. This is better done using ATP before a new attempt to induce VF is started, provided the patient tolerates the arrhythmia long enough to manually deliver ATP therapy.

High-voltage therapies are programmed according to the protocol used for induction. Usually, the ICD is allowed a maximum of two to three attempts with high-voltage therapy before the external defibrillator takes over. The first ICD therapy is programmed for the energy subjected to testing. Following therapies are programmed either for increasing energy or for maximum energy from the second therapy.

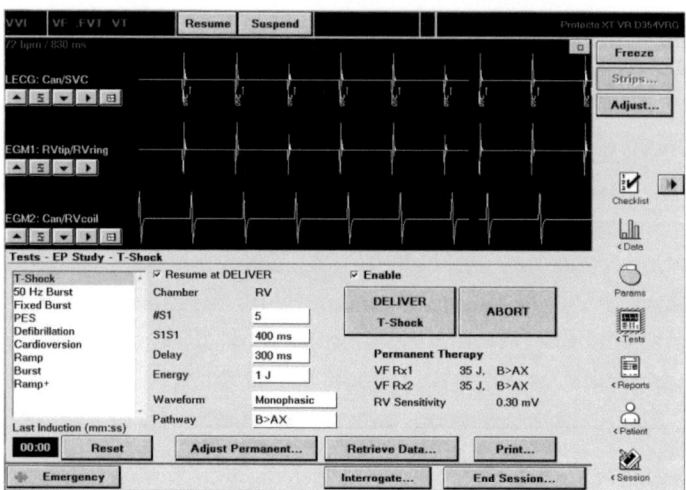

FIGURE 9.3 Induction menu from a Medtronic programmer model 2090.

When programming of the ICD has been done (and the external defibrillator connected and switched on), and all the staff is informed about the routines to be followed, induction of VF may be commenced. This is usually done from a specific programmer menu (EP menu or similar) where various induction protocols are available. The most commonly used options are T wave shock and 50 Hz burst.

T Wave Shock

This is, by far, the most commonly used induction method, based on the fact that a high-voltage pulse correctly timed to the T wave may induce ventricular fibrillation. The energy used should not exceed 1 J since higher energies decrease the chance of successful induction. The T wave shock protocol initiates a number of pacemaker pulses followed by a high-voltage pulse with a programmable delay to the last pacing pulse. A delay of 300 ms is usually a good starting point. If the first attempt is not successful at inducing the arrhythmia, a scanning program is initiated with alternating prolongation and shortening of the delay until VF is successfully induced. Changes of 20 ms may be sufficient. A scanning protocol may include the following sequence: 300 ms, 320 ms, 280 ms, 340 ms, 260 ms, etc.

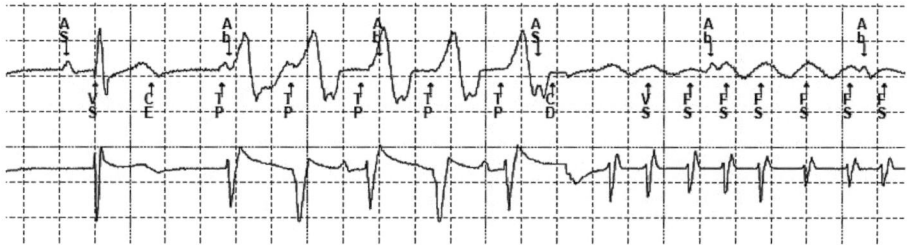

FIGURE 9.4 Induction using T wave shock. Note the number of pacemaker pulses (TP) preceding the T wave shock (CD = Charge Delivered).

If VT is induced instead of VF, no evaluation can be done concerning defibrillation energy. If possible, the VT is terminated by the use of ATP, after which a new attempt to induce VF can be made.

After successful induction and termination of VF, a waiting period of approximately five (5) minutes is advised before a new induction is attempted, in order to give time for recovery. To aid during implant, some programmers display a timer on the induction screen, showing the time since the last induction.

50 Hz

If repeated attempts to induce VF using T wave shock have failed, the method of induction may be switched to 50 Hz burst. This can be done from the programmer induction menu as well. Never deliver more than 10 seconds of 50 Hz at a time since the circulation stop initiated during the induction is added to the time it takes for the ICD to detect the arrhythmia, charge the capacitors, and deliver therapy. When the 50 Hz burst terminates, the ICD initiates detection in the same way as after induction using T wave shock.

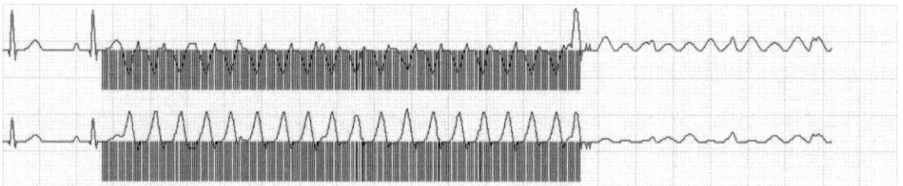

FIGURE 9.5 Induction using 50 Hz.

ULV and the VSM Test

In an attempt to cover all aspects of measuring defibrillation energy, I have chosen to include a description of the VSM (vulnerability safety margin) test as well. This test has the advantage of estimating DFT without taking the risks involved in induction of VF. The VSM test is based on studies showing that a minimum field strength over the whole myocardium is needed for successful defibrillation. This is called the upper limit of vulnerability (ULV) and uses the unit V/cm. If the defibrillation pulse allows for a field strength below the ULV in any part of the ventricle, VF may be re-induced in cells that are in the vulnerable phase when the energy is delivered. This is manifested by an isoelectric interval seen directly after the energy was delivered, which is then immediately followed by re-initiation of VF. ULV for human heart cells is approximately 4 V/cm for biphasic pulses, and approximately 6 V/cm for monophasic pulses. If the defibrillation pulse results in a field strength above ULV, it will lead to successful defibrillation.[10]

This is also the theory behind why induction using T wave shock should limit the shock energy to around 1 J. The energy needs to be high enough to initiate VF but needs to be kept below ULV in at least some parts of the myocardium. If T wave shock energy results in a field strength above ULV, VF will not be induced since the whole myocardium is activated simultaneously, not allowing for reentry circuits to form.

The theory behind the ULV test is that delivered energies that result in field strength below ULV may induce VF but can never result in defibrillation, while energies above ULV will not induce VF but will be enough for successful defibrillation. With this knowledge, it is possible to test safety margin for defibrillation without actually have to induce VF! This is done by delivering a T wave shock in the vulnerable phase of the T wave, with an energy that is above both the fibrillation threshold (to induce fibrillation) AND the ULV over the whole myocardium (usually three attempts at 15, 18 or 21 J). However, should ULV not be reached in any part of the myocardium, VF will be induced. The goal is to avoid induction, but it is important to understand that induction of VF is possible. If it can be shown that enough safety margin can be maintained to the ICD maximum deliverable energy—i.e., that a comparatively low energy in the T wave shock does not lead to induction of VF—the testing is stopped without having to induce VF.

---

[10] David L. Hayes, Samuel Asirvatham, Paul A. Friedman. *Cardiac Pacing, Defibrillation, and Resynchronization: A Clinical Approach*. Wiley-Blackwell 2008

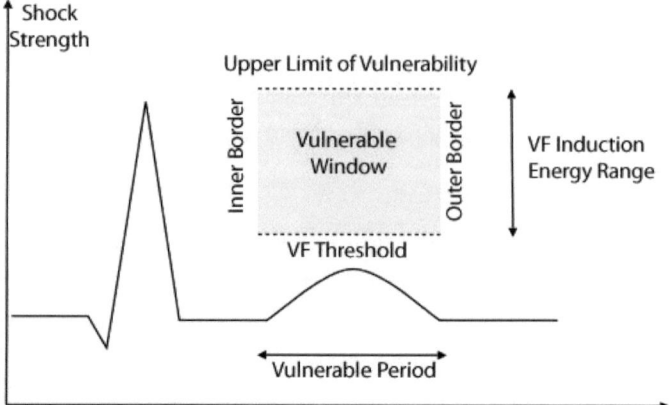

FIGURE 9.6 Window of vulnerability. For energies above or below the vulnerable window, VF induction will not be possible.

High DFT

When DFT seems to be high (normally defined as a safety margin of less than 10 J to the maximum energy of the ICD), we need to have strategies available to handle this situation. The first step is always to check all connections between the leads and the ICD to make sure that they are OK. This is done by a visual inspection of the connectors and by looking at the high-voltage impedances. If everything seems to be in order, the next step is to evaluate the position and the number of lead/s, and finally, a change of the pulse itself may be called for.

RV Lead Position

It is of utmost importance that the energy field built up between the high-voltage coils cover as much of the ventricular myocardium as possible. The position of the RV lead therefore plays an important role. The goal is to reach a position as apical as possible, and this is the first thing that should be checked if there is a problem with high DFT. Even small changes in lead position may have a substantial effect on DFT. If an apical lead position results in suboptimal values for sensing and/or pacing, the use of a separate pace/sense lead may be considered.

SVC

If the RV lead is in an apical position, the next step may be to consider how the other high-voltage leads affect the spread of the energy field over the myocardium. If a dual-coil lead is used, DFT is sometimes lower with the SVC coil disconnected (or, if possible, programmed to be inactive). This could be more effective in lowering DFT in patients with low high-voltage impedance ($< 40 \, \Omega$). Unfortunately, the use of dual-coil leads does not allow for a change in SVC coil position, which is possible if a separate SVC coil is used. If a single-coil lead is used, the addition of an SVC coil may be considered.

Active Can

Modern ICD systems use the can as one of the high-voltage poles. Some systems allow for the can to be disconnected as an active pole. This is especially useful in right-sided implantations since using the can as an active pole leads the energy away from the heart and increases DFT.

Addition of a Subcutaneous Lead

If the transvenous leads are optimized in position and number, only the addition of a subcutaneous lead (SQ lead) remains. This is done by tunneling the lead to a position just under the scapula laterally toward the spine. This procedure is done under general anesthesia.

Change of Pathway/Polarity

Except for changes in the lead system, there are some changes that may be made to the defibrillation pulse itself. These changes do not affect DFT as much as a change in the lead system but may be of some importance for selected individuals. One way to change the pulse is to change its pathway. In the most common pathway, the RV coil starts as cathode (−) during the first phase of the defibrillation pulse, but this may be reprogrammed to a reverse polarity with the RV lead as anode (+). This is often part of a programming strategy where the first defibrillation therapies are delivered with one polarity, which is then reversed for some of the last therapies.

Changes in Tilt/Pulse Width

Some systems allow for a change of the pulse appearance by reprogramming the tilt or pulse width. If DFT is high, reprogramming of tilt or pulse width may be considered. However, neither tilt nor pathway changes will result in a large change in DFT. To really make a difference, a change in the lead system to better cover the myocardium is often needed.

Right- or Left-Sided Implantation

An ICD is commonly implanted pectorally on the left side. This is the optimal position for the use of the active can and also creates fewer problems for the right-handed patient. However, there are some occasions when a right-sided implantation may be necessary—for example, if the vessels on the left side cannot be used for lead introduction (as in a lead replacement where the vessels on the left side are already used). A right-sided implantation should always be followed by DFT testing to check for optimal lead configurations and possible deactivation of the active can.

Programming for Shock Reduction and the Studies behind it

When programming an ICD, it is important to adapt the various parameters to the individual patient. Some of the things that need to be taken into consideration are:

- Is this a primary or secondary prevention patient?
- Are there known VTs that need treatment?
- What is the highest sinus rate?
- Does the patient have AT/AF? If so, what is the ventricular response (i.e., rate) during those arrhythmias?
- Is there an indication for brady-stimulation?

There are also some study results available that may be used as guides when choosing a final programming after the implantation. It is important that the programming strategy be well thought out and that all information about known arrhythmias be accounted for. This first setup of the device may very well make the difference between a patient who feels safe with the device and one who comes back to the emergency room with inappropriate/unnecessary high-voltage therapies. The latter often leads to much anxiety and even fear of the implanted device.

The studies most commonly referred to when discussing programming strategies are the following:

- PainFREE Rx and PainFREE Rx II
- PREPARE
- EMPIRIC
- ADVANCE III

A short summary of each study and its implications for programming strategy follows below.

PainFREE Rx and Rx II

These two studies investigated whether the number of high-voltage therapies may be safely decreased without an increased risk of syncope, accelerated arrhythmia, or sudden death, by treating faster ventricular arrhythmias (188–250 bpm) with ATP. The studies were published in 2001 and 2004 respectively and conclude that a vast majority of the episodes detected at rates > 188 bpm are VT (only 3% of the fast episodes in PainFREE Rx[11] and 10% in PainFREE Rx II[12] were true VF). Among the arrhythmias with a rate between 188 and 250 bpm, three out of four could be terminated by ATP (85% in PainFREE Rx and 72% in PainFREE Rx II). PainFREE Rx showed a syncope rate of 2%, which is in line with other studies. Acceleration of the arrhythmia could be seen in 4% of the episodes, which is not higher than in other ICD studies. The authors conclude that by programming two sequences of ATP (burst 88%, 8 pulses), it is possible to

---

[11] CIRCULATION 2001;104:796-801
[12] CIRCULATION 2004;110:2591-6

safely decrease the number of high-voltage therapies delivered. This leads not only to a decrease in morbidity but also to increased ICD longevity due to the small current drain needed to deliver ATP therapy. In PainFREE Rx II, the patients were randomized to either one sequence of ATP therapy and then high-voltage therapy or to high-voltage therapy as the first choice for VTs in the range of 188–250 bpm. The ATP group had a reduction of over 70% in the number of high-voltage therapies delivered, as well as higher scores for quality of life after twelve months. It is worth mentioning that modern ICD systems no longer need to be programmed as in PainFREE to achieve these results. The use of ATP during charge as standard programming simplifies programming in this regard.

Programming according to PainFREE RX II

Detection	Rate	Therapy
FVT via VF	188–250 bpm	RX1 = Burst, 8 pulses, 88%, 1 sequence
		RX2–RX6 = CV, 36 J

EMPIRIC

The EMPIRIC study was published in 2006 and was founded on the authors' concern that the ever-increasing number of ICD patients may lead to decreased quality of care, affecting safety and efficacy. To simplify programming procedures, they investigated whether an initial programming strategy with pre-set detection parameters and therapies may give the same results as manual individualized programming for each patient. EMPIRIC[13]

---

[13] J Am Coll Cardiol 2006;48:330-9

included 900 ICD patients with indications for primary or secondary prevention ICD treatment.

Programming according to EMPIRIC

Detection	Threshold	NID	Therapy
VF on	250 bpm	18/24	30 J x 6
FVT via VF	200 bpm	18/24	Burst (1 sequence), 30 J x 5
VT on	150 bpm	16	Burst (2), Ramp (1), 20 J, 30 J x 3

Discriminator

PR Logic on; AF/Afl, Sinus Tach

Programming strategy for the two study groups (empiric versus individualized) differed markedly, especially when looking at the VT zone, which was significantly lower (150 bpm) in the empiric group than for the control group. Hence, patients in the empiric group were more likely to receive therapy even for slower arrhythmias. Programming in the empiric group also included higher NID, more frequent use of sophisticated SVT discriminators, more use of ATP, and higher energy in the first high-voltage therapy. The EMPIRIC results showed that the empiric programming strategy used in the study was at least as safe and effective as individualized programming when it came to the number of high-voltage therapies delivered and time to first high-voltage therapy, as well as for syncope and mortality. In addition, the proportion of high-voltage therapies on slower VT episodes in the empiric group could be decreased due to more frequent usage of ATP. The conclusion from the EMPIRIC study is that a well-considered empiric programming oftentimes is at least as good as an individualized programming, which may facilitate the work in the ICD clinic.

PREPARE

The PREPARE study[14] (Primary Prevention Parameter Evaluation Study) was published in 2008 and focused on programming strategies for primary prevention ICD patients. The objective was to investigate whether a strategic programming of detection and therapy could decrease the number of high-voltage therapies delivered for VT/VF as well as for SVT. Seven hundred patients had a Medtronic ICD implanted and were followed for one year. The programming strategy was as follows:

- Only detection of fast arrhythmias (> 182 bpm)
- Only detection of sustained arrhythmias (NID 30/40)
- ATP as first therapy also for fast VT
- SVT discriminators activated
- First high-voltage therapy given at maximum energy

VF zone was programmed to > 250 bpm. This programming strategy resulted in a decrease in the total number of high-voltage therapies (compared to the control group) without increasing the risk for syncope or death and with a decreased morbidity.

---

[14] J Am Coll Cardiol 2008;52:541-50

Programming according to PREPARE

Detection	Rate	NID	Therapy
VF on	> 250 bpm	30/40	30-35 J
FVT via VF	182–250 bpm	30/40	1 sequence ATP, 30–35 J
VT monitor	167–181 bpm	32	None

Discriminator, single-chamber	Discriminator, dual-chamber
Wavelet on; SVT Limit = 200 bpm	PR Logic on; AF/Afl, Sinus Tach

ADVANCE III

ADVANCE III[15] was published in 2013 and included both primary and secondary prevention patients with ICD or CRT-D. The purpose of the study was to find out whether a longer detection time (higher NID) can safely decrease the number of high-voltage therapies. This had already been shown in PREPARE for primary prevention patients, but evidence was still lacking for secondary prevention patients. In this study, 1902 patients were randomized to either NID = 18/24 or NID = 30/40 and were followed for two years. The study showed a 37% reduction in the number of delivered therapies (high-voltage and ATP) for NID = 30/40, with no difference in mortality or arrhythmic syncope between study groups.

Programming according to ADVANCE III

Detection
NID = 30/40
ATP during Charging = on

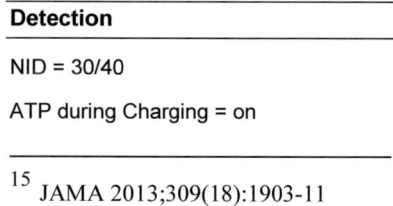

[15] JAMA 2013;309(18):1903-11

Diagnostics

An ICD may be seen as a computer continuously monitoring each heartbeat and delivering proper therapy when needed. It also has a large memory capacity where information is stored automatically for later viewing during follow-up. This information is commonly called *diagnostics*, although *data* is probably more correct since the diagnostic analysis is largely carried out by the physician/nurse responsible for the follow-up of the patient.

Collected and stored data may be divided into three categories:

- *Technical data about the system*, such as lead impedances, threshold values, battery data, charge times, etc.
- *Arrhythmia data* about detected arrhythmias and delivered therapies.
- *Other physiological data*, such as heart failure data and patient activity. Heart rate histograms, ventricular rate during atrial arrhythmias, and percentage of pacing in each chamber are often also available.

The diagnostic features in a modern ICD are extremely important and give us the opportunity to accurately evaluate technical function as well as the interaction between the ICD and the patient.

Technical Data

The ICD collects and stores data about its technical function (ICD and leads). Technical data is used to evaluate lead integrity as well as battery and capacitor status and represents an important part of ICD diagnostics.

Lead Impedance

The electrical resistance in the electrical circuit built up during stimulation of the heart is called lead impedance. However, this is not, as one may think, the impedance in the lead itself but rather the total impedance in the electrical circuit. The impedance, measured in Ohms, is commonly found between 400 and 1000 Ohms for low-voltage (pacemaker) leads, and between 40 and 70 Ohms for high-voltage leads. Dual-coil leads have somewhat lower high-voltage impedance than single-coil leads due to the larger surface area of the dual-coil.

The impedance value is affected by various factors, and lead construction plays a big part. Another factor is the lead position in the heart. A different position with the same lead in the same patient may result in a different impedance value. Different patients give different impedance values, and some changes in impedance values may be seen with various drugs, electrolyte imbalances, etc. Lead impedances for leads placed in the ventricle are generally higher than for those placed in the atrium, even if the same lead model is used. For pacing leads with a large percentage of pacing, the ICD current drain, and thus longevity, depends on the lead impedance. Higher impedance results in lower current drain for a given amplitude, as well as better longevity.

The most common problems seen in both ICD and pacemaker treatment are related to the leads. Lead dislocations are not uncommon during the first few weeks after implantation, and leads that have been implanted for a while may suffer from insulation damage or cable break. Since it is not possible to develop and produce leads that will function indefinitely in the hostile environment of the body, it is of high importance to continuously evaluate lead integrity. To discover an incipient lead failure before it results in symptoms or loss of treatment is desirable. Large variance over time, or continuously increasing/decreasing impedance, should always demand further investigation and possibly shorter follow-up intervals. Make it a habit to always check lead impedance measured values as well as impedance trends so as to increase the chances of early discovery of a failing lead.

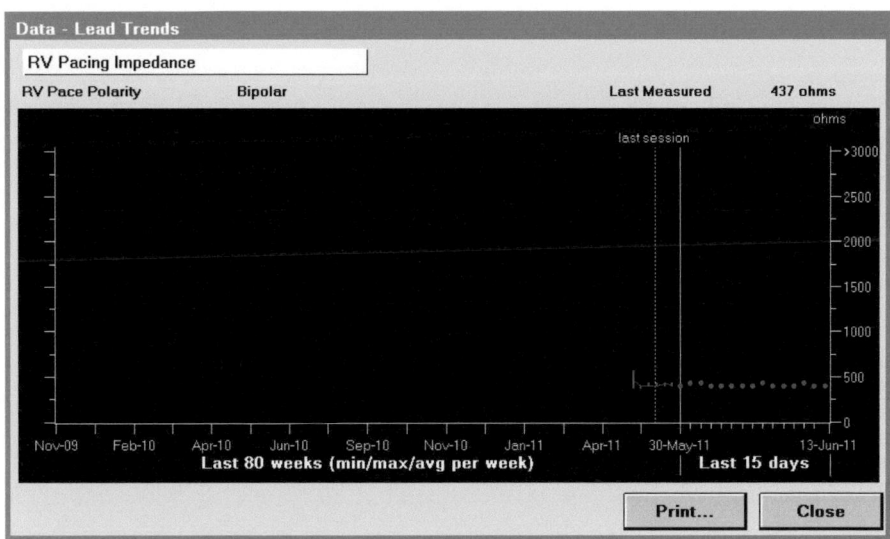

FIGURE 11.1 Example of a long-term lead impedance trend from the RV lead.

Changes in lead impedance for any of the pacing leads should always prompt further investigation of other diagnostics, such as threshold and sensing trends. Varying lead impedance is always a sign that something is wrong and so should never be overlooked. Evaluation of the ventricular pacing lead is particularly important since it is sensing on this lead that constitutes the foundation of ICD treatment. In failing leads it is not uncommon to see showers of noise originating from broken conductor wires in intermittent contact. These signals may be interpreted as VF by the ICD and result in repeatedly delivered inappropriate high-voltage therapy. This is a very serious condition and calls for immediate deactivation of the ICD system and replacement of the failing lead. Leads that were not correctly attached to the ICD connector may show a similar behavior. This is due to intermittent contact between the ICD and the lead and can only be solved by a reoperation where the lead is pulled out of the connector block and then reconnected correctly.

Impedance changes in the high-voltage leads are more difficult to evaluate but are no less important. A damage high-voltage lead may look fine up until the time that the patient needs therapy for a life-threatening arrhythmia. The system is then unable to deliver high-voltage therapy, which may lead to serious consequences for the patient.

Charge Time and Delivered Energy

Each time the high-voltage capacitors of the ICD are charged, the time to do so is measured. Charging of the capacitors is done after detection of an arrhythmia that calls for defibrillation, but also to reform capacitors or whenever a manual test charge is performed. The charge time is a reflection of capacitor performance. Longer charge time causes a longer delay in therapy and is a sign of suboptimal capacitor performance. In some systems, charge time increases with the age of the system and needs to be monitored closely. In other systems, charge time is relatively constant over the lifetime of the device, which is preferred. Since charge time constitutes a delay in therapy, it is important that it be as short as possible. Charge times of 10 seconds are desirable, but depending on the manufacturer, 12 seconds or more may need to be accepted. Charge time is measured by the ICD and is reported at interrogation.

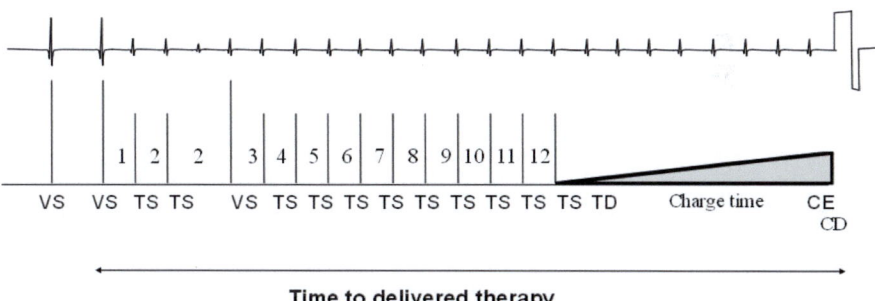

FIGURE 11.2 The time from arrhythmia start to delivered therapy depends on detection time (NID) and charge time.

After the capacitor has been charged and therapy has been delivered, it is also important to make sure that the full amount of energy has been delivered. If only a small part of the expected energy was delivered, a damaged lead may be suspected.

Therapy Sequence		
VF Rx 1 Defib	Energy	0.0 - 35.0 J
	Charge Time	6.80 sec
	Waveform	Biphasic
	Pathway	B>AX
	Delivered Energy	35.1 J
	Impedance	46 ohms

FIGURE 11.3 Printout from a Medtronic Protecta showing delivered energy, charge time, and high-voltage impedance.

Battery Data

Sooner or later, the day will come when the battery is discharged and the ICD needs to be replaced. To keep track of when a replacement needs to take place, battery status is checked at every follow-up. Depending on manufacturer and model, remaining longevity is presented in various ways. This may be checked through battery impedance and/or battery voltage. When the battery discharges, the internal impedance increases, causing the battery voltage to decrease. At a certain moment in time, these values will reach the levels pre-set by the manufacturer for a discharged battery, and a message will be shown on the programmer screen that the ICD has reached RRT (recommended replacement time). After RRT has been triggered, the battery usually will contain enough energy for another three months of service life at standard programming. Oftentimes, it will last even longer.

Projecting remaining longevity for an ICD is considerably more difficult than for a pacemaker since delivery of high-voltage therapies in an instant may decrease longevity by several months. The ICD battery also has a different chemistry than that of a pacemaker and often includes a plateau phase when battery voltage is constant even as the discharge process continues.

As battery longevity gets closer to RRT, it is common to perform follow-ups at shorter time intervals. Different clinics have different strategies for determining when a replacement should be done. Most ICDs will emit an audible sound when RRT is reached, and for patients connected to a wireless remote monitoring system, a message will be sent to the clinic that RRT is reached. The patient then needs to be scheduled for a replacement. For patients on remote monitoring that is not wireless, it is common to schedule more frequent transmissions closer to RRT in order to more carefully track the battery status and better plan for replacement.

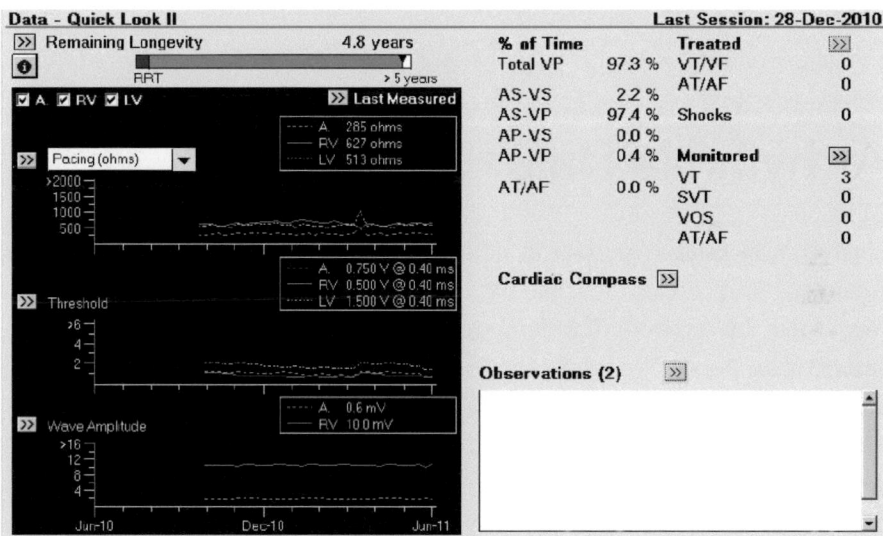

FIGURE 11.4 Example of the Quick Look screen from a Medtronic Viva XT showing the projected remaining longevity in years.

Sensing Integrity Counter (SIC)

The sensing integrity counter, SIC, is a feature available only in Medtronic devices but is nevertheless described in this book since it may provide very helpful information in case of lead damage and sensing issues. The sensing integrity counter monitors and counts short, non-physiologic RR intervals (< 130 ms). Signals with coupling intervals this short are usually not physiologic but are rather caused by noise and should always prompt a careful evaluation of ventricular lead integrity. Although SIC registrations can be found to have a physiologic explanation from time to time, the most common reason for high SIC count is some kind of oversensing that may very soon result in inappropriate high-voltage therapy unless necessary measures are taken. See also the chapter "Troubleshooting."

Arrhythmia Data

During ICD follow-up, stored data about possible arrhythmias and their treatment play a central role. By collecting and storing information that may later be viewed, the ICD provides the follow-up physician with information about each arrhythmia episode to help judging whether ICD reaction was appropriate or not. Was detection correct? Was the therapy delivered optimal for this arrhythmia? Was the first delivered therapy successful? Did the arrhythmia accelerate due to the delivered therapy? By viewing all stored episodes, possible sensing issues may be detected, such as T wave oversensing or lead noise from a broken lead.

EGM Episodes and Markers

To facilitate evaluation of all arrhythmia episodes, the ICD stores EGM signals as well as markers for the episode. The number of episodes that can be stored in the ICD memory differs between models but is significantly larger for ICDs than for pacemakers. Commonly, EGM is stored from two or more separate channels—for example, RV bipolar, RA bipolar, or an extracardiac registration such as can-to-SVC. Extracardiac tracings may be particularly useful when trying to differentiate between SVT and VT since this configuration also will provide information about morphology (broader QRS, for example) that may be more difficult to see in a bipolar registration. The EGM tracings will be followed by a marker channel that provides information about every single event. During follow-up, each episode should be viewed to assess the following:

- Was this a clinical arrhythmia or some kind of oversensing? What can be done to correct possible oversensing?
- Was this a ventricular arrhythmia that needed to be treated, or an SVT? In case of inappropriate therapy delivered on SVT, the discriminators should be evaluated and measures taken in order to avoid similar problems in the future.
- What was the starting mechanism? Can anything be done to prevent this trigger in the future? Reprogramming? Drugs?
- Was the arrhythmia correctly detected? Were all signals sensed?
- Was the optimal therapy delivered? Was high-voltage therapy delivered even though ATP could have been successful?
- Was the delivered therapy successful? Was the arrhythmia terminated? Accelerated?

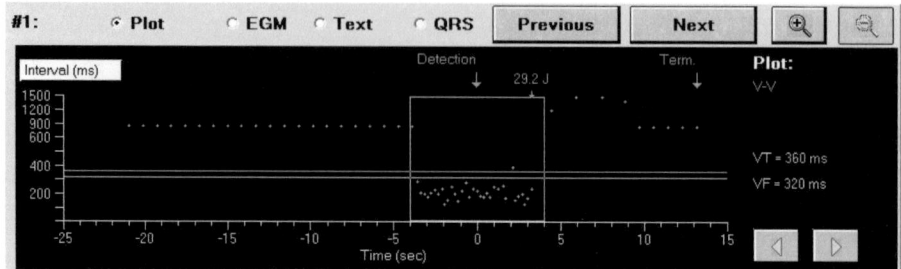

FIGURE 11.5 Arrhythmia plot from a Medtronic ICD showing VF with defibrillation and conversion to sinus rhythm.

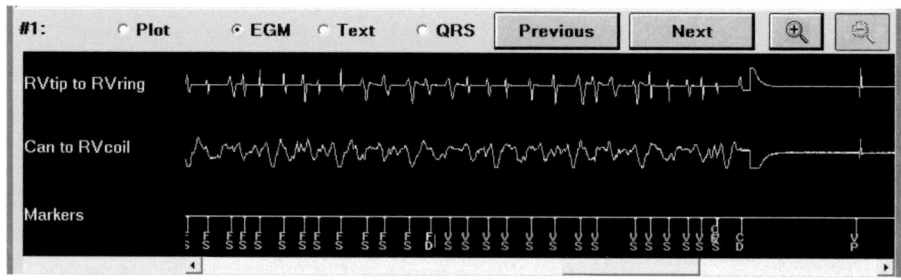

FIGURE 11.6 Example of EGM and marker channel during ventricular fibrillation. Note the FD (fibrillation detected) and CD (charge delivered) markers.

Arrhythmia Trends

Apart from studying the individual arrhythmias, it is also of interest to get an overview of the full arrhythmia burden. This is also true for atrial arrhythmias that may occur more or less frequently. Different systems have different trends and/or counters to provide information about when, how often, and how long the arrhythmias occur. Overviews may be available for what time of the day arrhythmias are most likely to start, about atrial arrhythmia burden, and also whether short episodes of VT (non-sustained VT) that do not lead to therapy are common.

Data - Counters				
○ **VT/VF Episodes**		○ **VT/VF Rx**		● **AT/AF Episodes**
		Prior Session 02-Apr-2011 to 06-Apr-2011		Last Session 06-Apr-2011 to 08-Apr-2011
AT/AF Summary				
% of Time AT/AF		7.9 %		12.6 % ↑
Average AT/AF time/day		1.9 hours/day		3.0 hours/day ↑
Monitored AT/AF Episodes		0.7 per day		0.5 per day ↓
Treated AT/AF Episodes		0.0 per day		0.0 per day
Pace-Terminated Episodes		0.0 %		0.0 %
% of Time Atrial Pacing		9.0 %		56.8 % ↑
% of Time Atrial Intervention		0.0 %		0.0 %
AT-NS (>6 beats)		0.5 per day		2.0 per day ↑
Since Last Session 06-Apr-2011 to 08-Apr-2011				
AT/AF Durations	**Episodes**	**AT/AF Start Times**	**Episodes**	
>72 hr	0	09:00 - 12:00	0	
48 hr to 72 hr	0	12:00 - 15:00	0	
24 hr to 48 hr	0	15:00 - 18:00	0	
12 hr to 24 hr	0	18:00 - 21:00	0	
4 hr to 12 hr	1	21:00 - 00:00	0	
1 hr to 4 hr	0	00:00 - 03:00	4	
10 min to 1 hr	0	03:00 - 06:00	1	
1 min to 10 min	0	06:00 - 09:00	0	
<1 min	4			

FIGURE 11.7 Trend data for atrial arrhythmias in a Medtronic Protecta XT.

Other Physiological Data

Beside arrhythmia data and information about the technical performance of the system, other diagnostic features are commonly available—for example, atrial and ventricular rate distribution, AV conduction, percentage of pacing in each chamber, and a number of heart failure parameters. Many of these functions are also found in modern pacemakers and, if used to do pacemaker follow-up, are easily recognized.

Rate Histograms

In the mid-1980s, the first pacemakers became available that could not only give therapy but also had the ability to collect data that could later be viewed by the use of a simple programmer. One of the very first diagnostic features in these devices was the rate histogram. For the first time it was possible to see at what rates the heart was beating, and at what rates the pacemaker was delivering therapies. Even though the rate histogram has been available for a long time, it is an important feature in modern devices that may be used to guide programming of the ICD. By viewing the histograms, important information about heart rates during exercise may be obtained, which is of interest when defining detection zones and for evaluation of chronotropic competence.

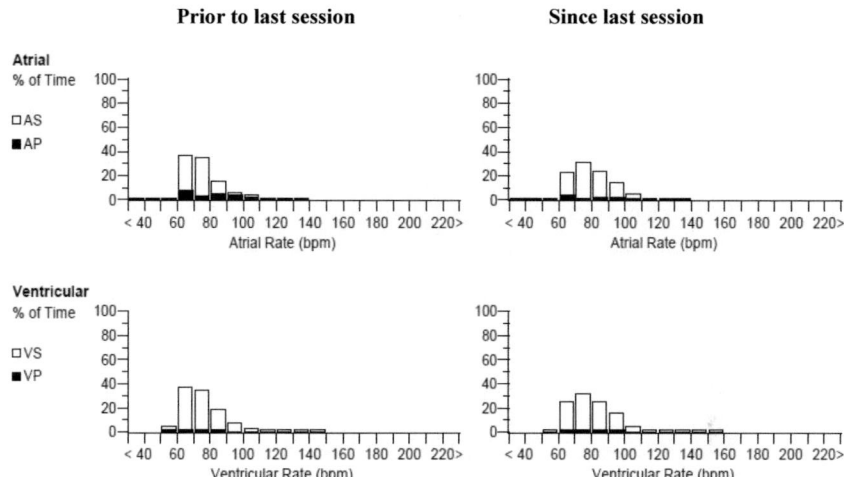

FIGURE 11.8 Example of a rate histogram report from a Medtronic Virtuoso DR. Histograms to the left are registered from the previous follow-up to the one before that, while histograms to the right are registered since the last session.

Stimulation Counters

Since a modern ICD also includes advanced pacemaker algorithms, diagnostics for those features need to be available as well. Since atrial and ventricular stimulation may account for a large portion of the energy consumed, and hence strongly affect longevity, it is important to know the amount of stimulation. It is also important to know whether the patient is pacemaker dependent and whether a sensor function for rate response needs to be activated to facilitate exercise. Many of the drugs regularly taken by this patient group depress the heart's ability to increase its rate, and rate response is sometimes well motivated. Stimulation counters provide information about the amount of pacing in the atrium and the ventricle in various combinations and, by doing so, also provide information about the AV conduction system.

% of Time	
Total VP	2.5 %
AS-VS	38.3 %
AS-VP	2.4 %
AP-VS	59.1 %
AP-VP	0.1 %

FIGURE 11.9 Example of event counters. Heart rhythm was spontaneous in 38.3% of events (AS-VS). Atrial stimulation occurred in 59.2% of events and ventricular stimulation in 2.5%.

Heart Failure Data

The majority of ICD patients suffer from heart failure, which makes it desirable for the ICD to also monitor heart failure status. This area is still under development, and it is very likely that in the future we will see even more sophisticated ways to monitor heart failure in the ICDs as well as in separate devices developed for this purpose alone.

The built-in heart failure diagnostics may monitor, for example, intra-thoracic impedance. This measurement is based on the fact that with increasing heart failure, more fluid accumulates in the lungs, which results in lower intra-thoracic impedance. Conversely, less fluid accumulation (drier lungs) results in higher impedance. These measurements may be connected to an audible alarm for the patient to hear, or to an automatic alarm sent via a remote monitoring system to the clinic, to draw attention to a deteriorating heart status. In this way, an early warning can be achieved, often before symptoms occur, and treatment with, for example, an increased dosage of diuretics can be administered. Examples of this kind of feature include Medtronic OptiVol™ and St. Jude Medical's CorVue™.

Other available heart failure diagnostics include:

- Measuring patient activity via the rate response sensor. With deteriorating heart failure, the patient normally becomes less active due to the other heart failure symptoms.
- Measuring mean heart rate night/day. Increasing mean heart rate is a sign of deteriorating heart failure.
- Measuring heart rate variability (HRV), which tends to decrease with deteriorating heart failure.

Follow-Up

Follow-up for an ICD is done either as a physical visit to the hospital's ICD clinic or as a remote follow-up where data is transmitted from the device to the clinic over the internet. Follow-up can be done at scheduled intervals (for example, every three or six months), or acutely, as when high-voltage therapy has been delivered. The follow-up may be divided into a technical part, checking the technical aspects of the ICD, and a clinical part with evaluation of arrhythmias, changes in medications, etc. The technical check-up does not essentially differ from that of a pacemaker. For arrhythmia-free patients, the clinical evaluation can be performed in a short time, but for patient with arrhythmias and/or delivered therapies, this part of the follow-up may be both time-consuming and require in-depth knowledge of the algorithms of the implanted ICD. Inappropriate therapies especially require extra time for troubleshooting and taking care of possible patient anxiety. It is highly recommended that the ICD clinic establish cooperation with a cognitive behavioral therapist who understands the possible psychological consequences of delivered high-voltage therapy (correct as well as inappropriate).

Technical Check-Up

As mentioned earlier, the technical part of ICD follow-up doesn't differ much from that of a pacemaker. However, it may be wise to use a pre-defined checklist to ensure that all tasks are done. An example of a task list follows below.

1. Interrogate the ICD and check the patient's current heart rhythm on ECG. Is everything normal? Can any unexpected markers be seen suggesting oversensing? Are all P waves/R waves being sensed correctly?
2. View the EGM signals. Sensed complexes should be narrow and not vary too much in amplitude, no signs of T wave oversensing should be found, EGM baseline should be free from noise that may indicate lead damage.
3. Perform an atrial/ventricular sensing test. Are the amplitudes acceptable?
4. Perform an atrial/ventricular threshold test and compare the results to the programmed output (pulse amplitude and pulse width). Is the safety margin large enough?
5. Evaluate lead impedance trends. Large impedance variations, or a continual increase/decrease, may be signs of upcoming lead problems. If available, check SIC counts for further indications of a failing lead.
6. Check battery data and estimate remaining longevity to RRT (recommended replacement time). A device manual may be necessary to do so.
7. Check capacitor charge time from the last charge. Is the value within the manufacturer's specification?

Clinical Check-Up

A modern ICD has the capability to store large amounts of data, including information about the patient's clinical status. For example, information is stored about ventricular arrhythmias and delivered therapies, atrial arrhythmias (arrhythmia burden, length of episodes, ventricular rate during atrial arrhythmia, start times, etc.), number of PVCs, mean heart rates during day/night, and possibly also information about heart failure status such as intra-thoracic impedance (for example, Medtronic OptiVol or St. Jude Medical CorVue).

For the clinical part of the follow-up as well, it may be wise to use a checklist to ensure that nothing is forgotten. An example of a checklist follows below.

1. Evaluate stored ventricular arrhythmias. Is the system functioning as intended? Are correct therapies being delivered? Are the first delivered therapies successful? If not, can changes be made for better success? Are detected arrhythmias clinical arrhythmias that need therapy? If not, what needs to be changed? Are there monitored episodes where therapy was called for?
2. Evaluate stored atrial arrhythmias. Is sensing correct? Is the ICD interpretation of the arrhythmia correct? For how long are the episodes going on? Anticoagulants? Rhythm or rate regulation?
3. Check the other diagnostics. Are there any changes from the last session? What is the rate distribution? Chronotropic incompetence? Is the ventricle unnecessarily stimulated? Anything else that needs to be changed in the programming?

Early ICD systems were often checked every three months, but today it is more common to check on ICD patients every six months. If the patient is on remote monitoring, is stable, and regularly sees a heart failure physician or the primary care unit, ICD follow-up visits may be restricted to once per year.

Remote Follow-Up

Remote ICD follow-ups have been performed in the U.S. since 2002. Patients with access to remote follow-up do not need to visit the ICD clinic to have their devices checked. This may instead be done from their homes by using a transmitting device (monitor), connected to the telephone line or the GSM network, which reads and transmits the data from the implanted device. Data is then reviewed at the ICD clinic, and the patient only has to visit the clinic if something needs to be changed. Remote follow-up offers several advantages for the patient:

- Time-saving: working patients do not have to take the day off and come to the hospital for follow-up, and for elderly patients who need assistance to get to the hospital, their relatives don't have to take the day off.
- No cost for transportation or parking.
- Fragile patients can avoid stressful transportation.
- Children with bad experiences from the hospital environment can be checked from their homes, avoiding a stressful visit.

The number of patients being treated with an ICD is increasing, which leads to increased pressure on ICD follow-up clinics. Remote follow-up can help the health care system in a number of ways.

- Time-saving: less time is needed to perform a remote follow-up than to perform the follow-up with the patient in the clinic.
- Economically advantageous: studies show that remote follow-ups can be done at lower costs than patient follow-ups in the clinic.[16]
- Necessary troubleshooting and interpretation of diagnostic data may be done at leisure, and diagnosis and possible actions may be communicated with the patient when decided upon.
- Fewer unplanned visits: some unplanned visits from worried patients may be avoided if the transmitted data looks fine.
- When more frequent follow-ups are needed—for example, for battery check-ups closer to RRT, to more closely follow a suspect lead, or to evaluate changes in medication—these are performed faster and more easily with remote follow-up.

One condition that needs to be fulfilled for remote follow-ups to be successful is that the implanted device must be able to provide and transmit all necessary information needed to judge arrhythmia status, treated episodes, etc. Information about lead and battery status should also be transmitted, as well as other data that would have been available at an in-clinic visit.

---

[16] Europace 2008 Oct;10(10):1145-51

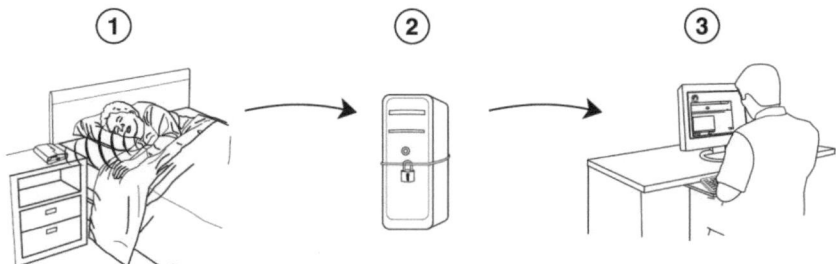

FIGURE 12.1 Wireless remote follow-up. The transmitting monitor is placed by the patient's bed (1) and transmits data automatically at scheduled time intervals. Should a problem be detected, the ICD will automatically transmit a message (alert) to the clinic together with the collected data. Data is sent to a central server (2), where the physician or nurse may log in to see the information from any computer with internet access (3).

Alerts

Most ICD models offer a possibility to activate alerts and send a warning if something is found that is out of the ordinary. This may be done in the form of an audio alarm (the ICD "beeps") for the patient to hear and to contact the ICD clinic, or by an automatic transmission from the remote monitor with data sent directly to the clinic. Alerts are commonly programmable and may include the following:

- Impedance alert if any of the lead impedances are out of range
- LIA (Medtronic lead integrity alert) if signs of lead failure are detected
- Battery alert when the battery reaches RRT
- Charge time alert for excessive charge times
- Therapy alert if more than one high-voltage therapy has been delivered in one episode

- Heart failure alert if a pre-defined limit has been reached by, for example, OptiVol

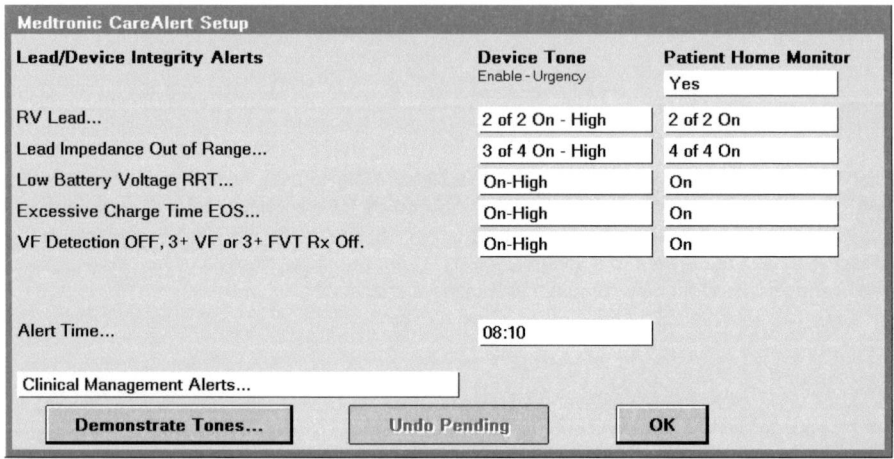

FIGURE 12.2 Example of a programmer screen to set ICD alert functions (Medtronic Protecta).

Deactivation

Although an ICD should almost always be switched on after implantation, there may be instances when deactivation of the device for shorter or longer periods of time is necessary. This is the case when there is an increased risk of inappropriate therapy, such as with broken leads causing oversensing, T wave oversensing, or during surgery where diathermy is used. ICD treatment may also be terminated if no longer favorable for the patient. This may be done in dying patients or in patients with other serious diseases with a short expected survival time, where sudden cardiac death may be more desirable.

For shorter deactivations, performed primarily during surgery when there is no programmer available, it is possible to deactivate the ICD by the use of a strong magnet. The magnet, which is of the same type used for pacemakers, is taped in place over the device during the whole procedure and thus keeps the ICD functions switched off until removed (the pacemaker functions, however, remain unaffected). A magnet may also be used when a patient receives repeated inappropriate high-voltage therapies and no programmer is available—for example, in the ambulance.

Different ICDs are deactivated in different ways, and it is important to know at least how to deactivate the models found in one's own clinic. A patient with a temporarily deactivated ICD should always be monitored, with close access to an external defibrillation if necessary, until the system can be safely reactivated.

Noise Sources

In the same way as a pacemaker, an ICD has various ways to prevent signals originating from outside of the heart from being sensed. This is achieved by signal filtering on the input sensing amplifier that only allows signals of the same frequency content as the P wave/R wave to pass undisturbed. Signals with different frequency contents are damped, resulting in remaining amplitudes too small to be sensed. However, it is not possible to completely keep all noise signals out and at the same time maintain a high sensitivity to the small signals that need to be sensed to correctly detect ventricular fibrillation. It is therefore important to know what noise sources an ICD patient needs to avoid. While a pacemaker patient may get dizzy and possibly faint when in contact with powerful noise sources, the ICD patient risks inappropriate high-voltage therapy, which is both painful and potentially dangerous.

When it comes to external sources of noise, the strength of the signal diminishes by the square distance. Hence, most noise sources will reach safe levels if the patient increases the distance from the source by two to four feet. The patient should be instructed to always increase the distance from a potential noise source or, if possible, switch it off if symptoms of dizziness, palpitations, or delivered high-voltage therapy should occur. It is uncommon that the ICD is more than temporarily affected, but in very strong fields, there is a risk for device "reset." This is a safety function that initiates when the ICD circuitry is affected by very strong electrical fields, resetting the ICD to a safety set of parameters decided by the manufacturer. The ICD may later be reprogrammed to its original settings by the use of a programmer.

New products are constantly being introduced to market, and it is therefore not possible to present a complete list of which ones may be used and which should be avoided. Smaller appliances may be brought by the patient to the clinic and tested under safe conditions with ICD detection switched off. Larger machinery is clearly more difficult to test, but the manufacturer of the appliance should be able to provide information about compatibility.

Below is a list of appliances that are known sources of noise and that may affect ICD function. *Note that this is **not** a complete list and that appliances not on the list may still be potentially dangerous for an ICD patient to be around.*

Home environment:

- Ignition systems in car or motorcycle engines, chainsaws, garden trimmers, etc.
- Electrical stimulators for muscle building or pain relief (TENS)
- Scales measuring body fat by sending an electrical current through the body
- Antennas for amateur radio transmitters and similar equipment
- Charging equipment for car batteries
- Generators
- Pneumatic compressors
- Electric welding machines
- Starter cables for cars

Hospital environment:

- TENS
- Muscle stimulators
- Irradiation therapy
- Diathermy
- MRI

Although this list is not complete, this is some of the equipment most commonly discussed. Unless a current is sent through the patient's body, a safety distance of one to two feet is usually enough, depending on the strength of the electric field. The author strongly advises against the use of chainsaws, both electrical and petrol engines, due to the serious consequences that may result from the delivery of high-voltage therapy while using the saw.

Troubleshooting

ICD troubleshooting may be needed for different reasons. Some of the more common ones are described in this chapter. Intermittent problems are always more difficult to analyze than permanent ones, but by spending some time on a more thorough evaluation of the stored data, it is often possible to find the information needed to make the right decision on what corrective action to take.

Lead Impedance

Many of the problems that may occur within the ICD system originate from one of its leads. There may be a problem with the lead itself (cable break, insulation damage) or a faulty connection between the lead and the ICD. These kinds of problems can often be revealed by measuring lead impedance. The ICD measures the impedance in the total electrical circuit for the chosen lead (not only the impedance of the cable itself), including that of the contact between the lead connector and the ICD and of the interface between the lead and the heart. There is a difference in "normal" lead impedance between lead models, and it is therefore important to be well acquainted with the lead types used in one's own clinic. High-voltage leads, with a large surface area, have significantly lower impedance than do pacing leads. Since impedance values vary by model, it is not possible to give a general recommendation on what is normal and what is not, but impedance values of 400–1000 Ohms are quite commonly seen on pacemaker (low-voltage) leads, while high-voltage leads (RV and SVC coils) commonly measure 40–80 Ohms. Even more important than the absolute value is the stability of the value. Some physiological variances can always be accepted, but larger variations are usually a sign that trouble is on the way. The same is true for leads with a continuous impedance increase or decrease. For pacing leads, it is important to check whether the changes in impedance are also affecting stimulation threshold or sensing. If a correlation between changes in impedance and changes in threshold or sensing can be found, this usually implies that there is a technical problem in the cable or connector. If no such correlation can be found, the reason for impedance change is more likely physiologic and may be found in the interface between the lead and the heart.

High impedance values are due to a disruption in the electrical circuit. This may be a break in the lead cable or a faulty connection between the lead and the ICD. When this happens in leads used for sensing, oversensing can often be seen as intermittent contact generates small electrical signals large enough to be picked up by the ICD. These problems are almost always intermittent and may be discovered as large variations in the impedance trend or as short episodes stored in the ICD as non-sustained VT. In ICDs from Medtronic, this phenomenon also manifests as high SIC counts. If oversensing is persistent, it may result in inappropriate therapy.

Integrity problems of high-voltage leads are often more difficult to discover. Modern ICDs measure lead impedance even on high-voltage leads with low amplitude, sub-threshold pulses. This measuring method gives a good idea about low-voltage lead function, but is unfortunately not as safe for high-voltage leads. To correctly measure lead integrity for high-voltage delivery, the measuring pulse needs to be of the same strength as that used for defibrillation. Since this is not possible due to the pain that it would cause the patient, problems with the high-voltage leads are more difficult to evaluate. The first sign of a problem may be when high-voltage therapy is needed but cannot be delivered due to lead failure.

When troubleshooting instable lead impedances, the following steps may be indicated:

- Repeated impedance measurements in various patient postures such as lying down, sitting, arms stretched over the head, etc.
- Manual provocation around the ICD pocket during repeated impedance measurements.
- X-ray or fluoroscopy to check cable and connectors (it is often possible to see whether the connector is completely pushed into the connector block), especially on recently implanted systems.
- X-ray of the lead path from the device to the heart. Lead damage is often found to be caused by compression of the lead body between the clavicle and the first rib, known as a subclavian crush.

Large variations in lead impedance always call for a careful evaluation and often cannot be solved without surgery.

In slower but persistent increases/decreases in lead impedance, it is usually more difficult to find the cause. The following may be considered:

- Physiologic changes in the tissue around the lead tip caused by progressive heart disease, or by the lead tip itself. A lead with too much tension caused by a poor anchoring of the lead to the vessel, for example, may cause stress to the tissue in contact with the lead tip, leading to fibrosis. A stretched lead may be seen using an X-ray.

- Some lead models have a tendency to drift in impedance over time. Discuss with the manufacturer what is acceptable for the model in question. Usually, other measured parameters will indicate when it is time to abandon the lead. If the threshold is low and sensing is fine, slowly drifting impedances may be accepted within reasonable limits.

Oversensing

Oversensing usually manifests itself in one out of two ways; silent oversensing detected at follow-up without preceding patient symptoms, and oversensing that has triggered therapy (usually defibrillation) with the patient seeking acute hospital care. Oversensing should always be taken seriously, especially if the patient has received inappropriate therapy, and should always lead to careful evaluation. Until the problem is solved, arrhythmia detection is switched off, and the patient is monitored in the hospital.

T Wave Oversensing

T wave oversensing (TWOS) is a well-known problem for ICD patients that may lead to detection and inappropriate therapy at rates as low as half the detection rate. As described earlier, there are a few different reasons why this problem occurs. If oversensing occurs during exercise and is caused by pathological T wave changes due to ischemia but with normal

R wave amplitudes, even repositioning of the lead may prove to be unsuccessful at solving the problem. Manufacturers have various solutions that may be tried out:

- If the ICD has an algorithm to discriminate T waves, it should, of course, be switched on.
- For ICDs with programmable sensing configuration, sensing polarity may be changed from bipolar to integrated. However, it is important to make sure that the R wave is still of acceptable amplitude with the new configuration.
- For ICDs with programmable decay delay, this may be prolonged to avoid sensing of the T wave. However, it is important to remember that a longer blanking/decay delay will increase the risk of undersensing of fast arrhythmias.
- For ICDs with programmable start value for sensing (St. Jude Medical Threshold Start) as a percentage, this value may be increased to make sensing less sensitive directly after the QRS complex. However, this may have negative effects on the ICD's ability to detect true arrhythmias.

For patients with T wave oversensing due to diminishing R wave amplitudes, the strategies above can also be used, with the addition that if R wave amplitude is low enough to jeopardize arrhythmia detection (uncommon), or if the problem is persistent, repositioning of the lead or an additional pace/sense lead is necessary. To rely solely on TWOS-rejecting algorithms may prove too optimistic.

Regardless of what measures have been taken, it is mandatory to have patients perform an exercise test before detection is reactivated. Since the problem doesn't reveal itself at rest, an exercise test with the programmer head placed over the device for continuous monitoring of the sense markers is needed. ICD detection should be switched off during the whole test. If no oversensing can be noted, detection may be switched on. It is common for the patient to feel anxious about performing strenuous activities similar to the one causing the inappropriate therapy. The exercise test has the potential to lessen anxiety since it gives the patient a chance to exercise in a safe environment. For patients in whom strong anxiety remains, referral to a cognitive behavioral therapist may be indicated.

P Wave Oversensing

When programmed for integrated sensing polarity, the ICD measures the difference in potential between RV tip and RV coil. For this to work safely, it is important that the RV coil not protrude into the atrium. If the coil is too long or not placed apically enough, P waves may be sensed on the ventricular channel, possibly leading to detection and inappropriate therapy.

- Reprogramming of sensing polarity from integrated to bipolar will solve the problem. However, not all leads/devices offer this solution, which may make reoperation necessary.
- Reprogramming of sensitivity may in rare cases prove useful. Unfortunately, the P wave falls at the part of the heart cycle where the ICD has the highest sensitivity (just before the next R wave).
- Repositioning of the lead where the coil is pushed down into the ventricle as far as possible may work.

Lead Noise

ICD lead failures are more common than pacing lead failures. This is partly due to the more complex design of the ICD lead, but the fact that development of the ICD lead is still ongoing also plays a part. Thinner leads call for new materials, smaller cans for new connector standards, and possible flaws in the design are usually not discovered until after several years of implant. This is unfortunate, but it is a reality we will have to deal with for many years to come. Every clinic needs to keep track of which leads need more attention, as well as the latest recommendations for those leads.

As described earlier, a failing lead may show various failure mechanisms. The mechanism responsible for oversensing and possibly inappropriate therapy is conductor break in any of the conductors involved in sensing. Each conductor is constructed from thinner parts. If any of those parts fracture, intermittent contact between the fracture surfaces may occur, causing showers of electrical signals that may be detected by the ICD sensing circuits. If the signals are sustained, ICD criteria for detection may be fulfilled and therapy will be delivered. It is not uncommon for there to be repeatedly delivered therapies, which may be very traumatic for the patient. Unfortunately, the only solution to this problem is a lead change. However, there are some programming strategies that decrease the risk of inappropriate therapy should lead fracture occur. None of these are to be seen as permanent solutions, but they do increase the chances for early discovery of the problem before inappropriate therapy has been delivered. This is especially true for patients connected to wireless remote monitoring where an automatic alarm is generated if signs of a failure are detected. The patient can then be called in to the clinic to check the system and take appropriate measures.

Programming strategies to decrease the risk of inappropriate therapy due to lead fracture include:

- Increased detection time or NID (30/40). Showers of noise are often intermittent, and a longer detection time has the potential to allow the signals to cease before the detection criterion is met.
- Specific algorithms (discriminators) to detect lead noise and withhold detection.
- Medtronic LIA (lead integrity alert), which actively looks for signs of lead failure. If LIA criteria are met, the VF NID is automatically changed to 30/40, an audible alert is initiated, and a CareLink (remote monitoring) alert is transmitted to the clinic.
- Wireless remote monitoring will shorten the time from lead failure to physician's awareness. Then the patient may be called in for a check-up and have detection switched off, and actions can be taken to solve the problem before inappropriate therapy has been delivered.

External Noise

This is a relatively uncommon form of oversensing and is often found in association with water. Water is generally a good conductor for electrical current and increases the risk of leaked current being conducted through the patient's body. If this happens, it is important to find out where the patient was and what he was doing at the time the oversensing took place. If the problem cannot be solved, the patient should avoid this activity/place in the future.

No Therapy Delivered

Fortunately, this is a very uncommon problem but may also be the one most serious for the ICD patient. It is easy to understand that if the ICD does not succeed at delivering therapy on a clinical VF, there is a high likelihood that the patient will die. It is therefore not sure that there will be a second chance to correct, for example, a suboptimal programming of the device.

There are various reasons why an ICD may not deliver therapy when an arrhythmia occurs:

- Incorrect programming of the device, detection set to off, no therapies activated.
- The ICD has reached EOS (end of service) and is no longer able to deliver therapy due to a discharged battery.
- Technical malfunction of the ICD or its leads. In the case of a short-circuited high-voltage lead, some ICDs inhibit therapy since it would only destroy the ICD and not send energy to the heart.
- The ICD misjudged the rhythm. If this is the case, it is likely one of the discriminators misinterpreted the rhythm to be something other than VT/VF (for example, SVT). Since these algorithms are often of a complex nature, it may be necessary to contact the manufacturer for advice on what went wrong. Until the problem is solved, the patient should be monitored in the hospital.

Inappropriate Therapy due to SVT

SVT misinterpreted as VT is the most common reason for inappropriate therapy. In the "Discriminators" chapter, various algorithms were discussed that help discriminate between SVT and VT when rate alone is not enough. Should any of the discriminators be switched on? Should a discriminator that is presently switched on be switched off?

Here are some solutions to be considered to avoid inappropriate therapy due to SVT:

- The most common reason why a discriminator is not working is simply that it is not allowed to do its job! These algorithms are always subject to a rate limit; either there is a programmable rate over which the discriminators are not allowed to work, or the discriminators are not allowed to work in the highest detection zone. The reason for this limitation is, of course, that we cannot afford to risk a discriminator making the wrong decision and withholding therapy for a fast and potentially serious arrhythmia. However, oftentimes by setting the SVT limit too low, we don't allow enough room for the discriminators to work. This leads to inappropriate therapy on SVT that could have been avoided had the discriminators been allowed to do their jobs. In some devices (e.g., Medtronic Protecta), this has been solved by having the value for the SVT limit nominally set to 260 ms (231 bpm), which, according to SCD-HeFT, covers 99% of all SVTs.
- When programming the detection zones, the patient's intrinsic (sinus) rhythm needs to be taken into account. If possible, the lower rate limit for detection should be programmed above the

patient's maximum sinus rate. If this is not possible (high sinus rate and slow VT), the use of discriminators is the only solution.

- For patients with rapidly conducted AF, a morphologic discriminator is recommended. If such an algorithm is not available, or if it is not feasible due to, for example, rate-dependent bundle branch block, stability is the second best choice. However, at very fast conducted ventricular rates, the intervals tend to be relatively stable and the stability discriminator may mistake the rhythm for VT. In dual-chamber ICDs, possible algorithms for AV analysis should be switched on.
- For other types of SVT with stable AV conduction (1:1 flutter), morphology is the only discriminator that may be of help.

Sensing Integrity Counter, SIC

This is a specific function in Medtronic ICDs only that counts the number of sensed, very short, non-physiological intervals (< 130 ms). During normal function and bipolar sensing, the SIC counts are usually zero. In integrated sensing, this number may increase to around 100 per month due to the slightly higher occurrence of oversensing in this configuration. The SIC counter is thus a tool to help discover possible lead fractures causing oversensing before they lead to inappropriate therapy. SIC counts may also have physiological explanations such as:

- P wave oversensing (in integrated sensing where the upper part of the RV coil is found in the atrium)
- T wave oversensing closely followed by a PVC (T wave over-sensing alone is not enough to trigger SIC counts since R-to-T intervals are longer than 130 ms)

- Double sensing of wide QRS complexes

Since correct sensing is extremely important in the ICD, unexpected SIC counts should always be thoroughly investigated. If no inappropriate therapy has been delivered, the following may be considered to investigate SIC root cause:

- Check the impedance trend and perform repeated lead impedance measurements, possibly also while manipulating the ICD pocket, to discover non-physiologic impedance variations. Large variations between measurements in patients with registered SIC counts is most probably a sign of lead failure. Monitor EGM signals and markers during manipulation of the pocket. Any sign of noise/oversensing?
- Evaluate all stored ventricular arrhythmia episodes. Lead noise is mostly intermittent and will most likely be found among the non-sustained VT registrations.
- Temporarily increase ventricular sensitivity (lower value in mV) to reveal intermittent oversensing of physiological signals. If no oversensing is observed, manipulation of the ICD pocket, or vigorous arm movements, may be used to provoke the problem.
- Look through all stored episodes of EGM and markers from both atrium and ventricle. Is there a physiologic reason for the SIC counts? Look for R-to-R intervals shorter than 130 ms.
- Use fluoroscopy to check the lead and its connection to the ICD. It is not always possible to see lead damage this way, but it is well worth a try. Check that the lead pin is pushed all the way into the ICD connector. Look for unnatural, sharp bends of the lead cable that may be signs of cable fracture. If integrated sensing is used, check that the RV coil does not reach into the atrium.

Programming Recommendations

Naturally, when programming an ICD, it is important to weigh the needs of the specific patient. Although there is no "one size fits all" in ICD programming, a standard set of parameter values may be used as a base that may then be adapted if needed. Below are recommendations for programming of the basic parameters of the ICD. *Note that every patient is unique and therefore may need special adaptations to the programmed parameter values.*

Parameter	Recommendations
Pacemaker Parameters	
Mode	Depending on indications for pacing: Patients with no need for pacing are programmed to VVI mode with a lower rate of 30 ppm. Patients with AV block and a need for ventricular stimulation are programmed to DDD mode (with or without rate response), and patients with sick sinus syndrome are programmed to AAIR or, more commonly, DDDR, preferably with algorithms to promote intrinsic AV conduction (for example, Medtronic MVP).
Amplitude/Pulse Width	Two times safety margin for amplitude or three times safety margin for pulse width, calculated from the measured threshold values. < 2 V and > 1 ms are used

less often, with the exception of atrial amplitudes where < 2 V may be used, and on high thresholds where pulse widths > 1 ms may be used to increase safety margin. Until the first follow-up six to eight weeks after implantation, a higher safety margin is used. For ICDs with automatic threshold measurements and adaption of output, these features are switched on.

Sensitivity

For bipolar sensing, a sensitivity of 0.3 mV is commonly used for both atrium and ventricle. For patients with TWOS that may not be solved with TWOS discrimination, polarity, or decay delay, sensitivity may be changed to a higher value in mV (lower sensitivity). Sensitivity needs to be high enough to ensure correct sensing even during ventricular fibrillation with small amplitudes.

Lower Rate

For patients without need for pacemaker stimulation, VVI mode at a lower rate of 30 ppm is programmed. If pacemaker stimulation is indicated, lower rates between 50 and 70 ppm are commonly used. Higher rates result in shorter battery longevity. If a rate responsive mode (tracking or sensor function) is used, lower rate may be programmed to a lower value. 70 ppm may be chosen for patients with paroxysmal atrial fibrillation.

Upper Tracking Rate

Always programmed lower than the lowest detection zone. The formula "220 – age" used for pacemaker patients is usually not applicable on ICD patients who, due to more severe heart failure and more medications, neither should be nor are able to reach rates that high. UTR of 120–130 ppm is common.

AV Delay

For heart failure patients, intrinsic AV conduction should be promoted. If ventricular stimulation is indicated, a normal PQ delay is desirable.

SAV: commonly 150–170 ms in AV block patients. Longer if intrinsic AV conduction can be promoted. SAV is programmed approximately 30 ms shorter than PAV if no significant spike-P is noted.

PAV: commonly 180–200 ms in AV block patients. Longer if intrinsic AV conduction can be promoted. PAV is programmed approximately 30 ms longer than SAV if

172

no significant spike-P is noted. If a long spike-P is observed, the PAV is prolonged by the spike-P interval.

RV Polarity	Dependent upon ICD system. Bipolar is more common. Integrated sensing is exclusively used by some manufacturers and may be used if problems occur with TWOS or diminishing R waves.
PVARP and PVAB	PVARP and PVAB are used for the pacemaker part of the ICD but allow for sensing and detection of arrhythmias. PVAB is programmed to cover possible FFRW. PVARP needs to cover retrograde P waves, if present. Common values are PVARP = auto or 220–250 ms, and PVAB = 150 ms.

Detection

VF zone	Needs to be activated to allow for therapy. Must cover all rapid arrhythmias in need of high-voltage therapy. Commonly programmed to 320 ms (188 ppm).
FVT zone	Earlier used to get access to ATP therapies for rapid arrhythmias in VF zone. Less frequently used today as ATP during charging is often a better alternative.
VT zone	Used for patients with known VTs that are slower than the VF zone and for which ATP therapy is desirable. The lower rate limit for VT is programmed to the VT interval + 30 ms. For primary prevention patients, the VT zone is often replaced by a monitor zone.
Monitor Zone	Used to evaluate whether slower arrhythmias are present that may need treatment. No therapy is given on arrhythmias in the monitor zone.
VF Initial Detection	Since a majority of the arrhythmias also in the VF zone are VTs, it is wise not to deliver therapy immediately but to wait for a few seconds to see if the arrhythmia self-terminates. For ICDs with programmable NID, 30/40 is commonly used, but it is important to take into consideration the patient's cardiac performance. Is the arrhythmia well tolerated? NID = 30/40 corresponds to a detection time of < 10 seconds for arrhythmias with a rate of 188 ppm.

173

VF Re-detection	If the arrhythmia is re-detected after therapy has been delivered, the arrhythmia and possible circulatory arrest has been ongoing for quite a number of seconds already. It is therefore important that the next therapy be initiated as soon as possible. NID for re-detection is commonly programmed to 12/16, corresponding to a detection time of < 4 seconds.
VT Initial Detection	Arrhythmias in the VT zone are slower and normally better tolerated than arrhythmias in the VF zone. To minimize the risk of unnecessary therapy, and also the risk of accelerating the arrhythmia, the first therapy is delivered with some delay. For ICDs with programmable NID, NID = 16 is commonly used. The patient's ability to tolerate the arrhythmia determines how long the delay from arrhythmia start to delivery of therapy can be.
VT Re-detection	Time needs to be kept shorter than for initial detection since the arrhythmia has already been ongoing for a while. Common programming of NID for VT re-detection is NID = 12.

Discriminators

AV analysis	PR Logic, Rate Branch, SMART Detection, etc. These discriminators are normally on. For PRLogic "Other 1:1 SVT" is set to off until the first follow-up, when it may be switched on.
SVT Limit	The most common reason for inappropriate high-voltage therapy is that the discriminators are not allowed to do their job. For discriminators with proven clinical safety, analysis should be allowed even at relatively high rates, possibly with a timeout for sustained fast rates. For Medtronic PRLogic and Wavelet, an SVT limit of 260 ms (230 ppm) is normally chosen, which, according to SCD-HeFT, covers 99% of all SVTs. Some manufacturers only allow their discriminators to work in the VT zone.
Morphology	Normally switched on, especially for single-chamber ICDs.
Stability	This discriminator is used differently by the different manufacturers. For dual-chamber ICDs from Medtronic,

174

PRLogic is primarily used since this discriminator includes a regularity rule to discriminate AF. If possible, PRLogic is combined with Wavelet (morphology). Discriminators based on morphology most often have a higher specificity than stability and are therefore the better choice. For systems lacking other discriminators against AF, stability is switched on if needed.

Onset

Should be used with great care since the algorithm may miss exercise-induced VT and interpret the rhythm as sinus tachycardia, with possible serious consequences. If other discriminators are available, they should be primarily used. For example, the recommendation for Medtronic ICDs is to NOT use the onset discriminator.

RV Lead Noise

ICDs with this function should always have it activated.

TWOS

ICDs with this function should always have it activated.

Therapies

VF

All therapies activated at maximum energy.

VT

The first therapies are usually programmed to ATP and the last ones to high-voltage therapy. Different protocols are used for the ATP therapies. For example, Rx1 may be programmed to deliver burst therapy and Rx2 to deliver ramp therapy. 8 pulses at 88% is a common programming.

ATP during Charging

On. Usually burst with 8 pulses at 88%.

References

1   Mark S. Kremers, Stephen C. Hammill, Charles I. Berul, et al. *Heart Rhythm 2013;4:e59-e65*

2   Michael O. Sweeney, Andrea Natale, Kent J. Volosin, et al. Prospective Randomized Comparison of 50%/50% Versus 65%/65% Tilt Biphasic Waveform on Defibrillation in Humans. *PACE 2001;24:60-5*

3   Michael R. Gold, Mary R. Olsovsky, Michael A. Pelini, et al. Comparison of Single- and Dual-Coil Active Pectoral Defibrillation Lead Systems. *J Am Coll Cardiol 1998;31:1391-4*

4   Arthur J. Moss, Wojiech Zareba, W. Jackson Hall, et al. Prophylactic Implantation of a Defibrillator in Patients with Myocardial Infarction and Reduced Ejection Fraction. *N Engl J Med 2002;346:877-83*

5   Alan Kadish, Alan Dyer, James P. Daubert, et al. Prophylactic Defibrillator Implantation in Patients with Nonischemic Dilated Cardiomyopathy. *N Engl J Med 2004;350:2151-8*

6   Stefan H. Hohnloser, Karl Heinz Kuck, Paul Dorian, et al. Prophylactic Use of an Implantable Cardioverter-Defibrillator after

Myocardial Infarction. *N Engl J Med 2004;351:2481-8*

7   Gust H. Bardy, Kerry L. Lee, Daniel B. Mark, et al. Amiodarone or an Implantable Cardioverter-Defibrillator for Congestive Heart Failure. *N Engl J Med 2005;352:225-37*

8   Bruce L. Wilkoff, Volker Kühlkamp, Kent Volosin, et al. Critical Analysis of Dual-Chamber Implantable Cardioverter-Defibrillator Arrhythmia Detection. *Circulation 2001;103:381-6*

9   Charles D. Swerdlow, Bruce D. Gunderson, Kevin T. Ousdigian, et al. Downloadable Algorithm to Reduce Inappropriate Shocks Caused by Fractures of Implantable Cardioverter-Defibrillator Leads. *Circulation 2008;118:2122-29*

10   David L. Hayes, Samuel Asirvatham, Paul A. Friedman. *Cardiac Pacing, Defibrillation, and Resynchronization: A Clinical Approach.* Wiley-Blackwell2008

11   Mark S. Wathen, Michael O. Sweeney, Paul J. DeGroot, et al. Shock Reduction Using Antitachycardia Pacing for Spontaneous Rapid Ventricular Tachycardia in Patients With Coronary Artery Disease. *Circulation 2001;104:796-801*

12   Mark S. Wathen, Paul J. DeGroot, Michael O. Sweeney, et al. Prospective Randomized Multicenter Trial of Empirical Antitachycardia Pacing Versus Shocks for Spontaneous Rapid Ventricular Tachycardia in Patients With Implantable Cardioverter-Defibrillators: Pacing Fast Ventricular Tachycardia Reduces Shock Therapies (Pain FREE Rx II) Trial Results. *Circulation 2004;110:2591-96*

13   Bruce L. Wilkoff, Kevin T. Ousdigian, Laurence D. Sterns, et al. A Comparison of Empiric to Physician-Tailored Programming of Implantable Cardioverter-Defibrillators. *J Am Coll Cardiol 2006;48:330-9*

14   Bruce L. Wilkoff, Brian D. Williamson, Richard S. Stern, et al. Strategic Programming of Detection and Therapy Parameters in Implantable Cardioverter-Defibrillators Reduces Shocks in Primary Prevention Patients. *J Am Coll Cardiol 2008;52:541-50*

15   M. Gasparini, A. Proclemer, C. Klersy, et al. Effect of Long-Detection Interval vs Standard-Detection Interval for Implantable Cardioverter-Defibrillators on Antitachycardia Pacing and Shock Therapy. *JAMA 2013;309(18):1903-11*

16   M. J. Raatikainen, P. Uusimaa, M. M. van Ginneken, et al. Remote Monitoring of Implantable Cardioverter Defibrillator Patients: A Safe, Time-Saving, and Cost-Effective Means for Follow-up. *Europace 2008 Oct;10(10):1145-51*

Index

179

T

U

V

W

Z